# Alternative Social Agencies: Administrative Strategies

# Alternative Social Agencies: Administrative Strategies

Felice Davidson Perlmutter
Editor

The Haworth Press
New York • London

*Alternative Social Agencies: Administrative Strategies* has also been published as *Administration in Social Work*, Volume 12, Number 2 1988.



The Haworth Press, Inc., 12 West 32 Street, New York, NY 10001
EUROSPAN/Haworth, 3 Henrietta Street, London WC2E 8LU England

**LIBRARY OF CONGRESS**
**Library of Congress Cataloging-in-Publication Data**

Alternative social agencies : administrative strategies / Felice Davidson Perlmutter, editor.
p. cm.
"Has also been published as Administration in Social Work, Volume 12, Number 2, 1988" – T. p. verso.
Includes bibliographies.
ISBN 0-86656-783-6
1. Social work administration – United States. 2. Health services administration – United States. I. Perlmutter, Felice Davidson, 1931-
HV95.A65 1988
361'.0068 – dc19

88-4414
CIP

# Alternative Social Agencies: Administrative Strategies

## CONTENTS

## ABOUT THE GUEST EDITOR

**Felice Davidson Perlmutter, PhD,** Professor, School of Social Administration, Temple University, has written extensively in the area of social service administration. She has been instrumental in organizing a graduate social work program in administration which has received national recognition. She serves as a consultant and lecturer in the field.

# Alternative Social Agencies: Administrative Strategies

# Introduction

Felice Davidson Perlmutter, PhD

Alternative social agencies have become of increasing importance in the past two decades as they have been organized to meet a broad array of needs not met by older established agencies. While many of these agencies have struggled to be formed, few have managed to survive in a time when even more stable systems have been at risk. This issue of *Administration in Social Work* is designed to tell the story of a diverse set of successful alternative programs. Special attention is paid to the social problem being addressed, the mission of the agency, its policy and governance mechanisms, its target population, and its programs, from an administrative perspective.

The heuristic value of these articles should result in adaptations that may be possible in existing programs – adaptations and innovations which can revitalize our various social agencies, their various staffs, and board members.

Where possible, these articles can also help stimulate new services to be developed. However, this latter approach is more complicated and requires a particular set of conditions and an abundance of energy. The articles in this journal highlight some of the necessary elements for the planning and implementation of a new alternative agency. These include: (1) a committed group of initiators, (2) a clarity of mission, (3) a clearly explicated value framework, and (4) charismatic leadership for a sustained period of time. Finally, a new program requires committed staff members who are willing, and able, to earn minimal salaries as full-time or part-time professionals.

Each of the following articles demonstrates some of these unique elements from various settings in the public and voluntary, not-for-

---

Dr. Perlmutter, Guest Editor, is Professor, School of Social Administration, Temple University, Philadelphia, PA 19122. She is a member of the Editorial Board of *Administration in Social Work*.

 

profit, sectors. Both direct services and indirect services are presented.

Part 1 describes an array of direct services in the voluntary sector; while all four articles in this section are in health-related organizations and agencies, their structures and strategies are very diverse.

Principles of participatory democracy and self-management are explored by Allyson Young Schwartz, Eve Weiss Gottesman, and Felice Davidson Perlmutter in a case study of a very sophisticated agency which has managed to retain its commitment to these principles while adopting administrative mechanisms for survival. The deliberate evolution of its administrative strategies provides important insights.

"Shanti: An Alternative Response to the AIDS Crisis" is a discussion of an urgent response to an urgent problem. Nancy R. Hooyman, Karen I. Fredriksen, and Barbara Perlmutter describe a volunteer psychosocial support organization and the dilemmas it faces as it seeks to meet the ever-increasing community needs while also seeking to maintain and sustain its volunteer staff.

A very different perspective is provided by Burton Gummer as he discusses "The Hospice in Transition," an agency also concerned with caring for the dying. Gummer identifies the dilemmas faced by the hospice movement as it struggles to preserve its unique identity within the context of external influences.

Diane Kravetz and Linda E. Jones examine a grassroots effort which has developed into a successful state-wide program in Wisconsin. The relationship of the program as an "alternative" system, while embedded within a traditional agency, is of particular interest.

Part 2 focuses on public sector agencies which are not usually associated with alternative programs. Paul Keys describes an array of administrative strategies in a public human service agency in the Midwest which had long-range implications for that community. Attention is paid to politics, advocacy, entrepreneurship, and innovation.

The creation of an alternative work culture in a public service setting is described by Marie Weil. The role of charismatic leadership is highlighted here and serves to call attention to the unique opportunities for administrators who reflect Philip Selznick's concept of executive statesmanship.

Part 3 presents three articles which describe indirect services. An innovative administrative structure, Resources for Human Development, is the case under study by Robert Fishman. This agency serves the unusual function of facilitating and encouraging the development and implementation of new community programs. Its design is creative and should serve as a model for replication.

In a case study of alternative funds, Felice Davidson Perlmutter discusses four important organizations in Philadelphia which have developed in the past decade. While each of the four agencies are distinctive and meet very different needs, they form an important alternative to the traditional United Way. Their diverse strategies, carefully developed, merit careful consideration.

In a final article Felice Perlmutter discusses the implications for curriculum design at the graduate level which best meet the unique characteristics of alternative social agencies as well as the leadership requirements for this cohort. Special attention is paid to both class and field content.

Albert E. Wilkerson's Epilogue to this volume serves an important function as he highlights the theoretical issues and dilemmas inherent in alternative programs. He appropriately calls for research in this new arena which can provide data to help these agencies chart their future directions.

The intent of this special issue of *Administration in Social Work* is to help all of us involved in social administration to question our administrative practice and to struggle with new approaches which can best meet the needs of our present and/or potential constituencies.

# PART 1: DIRECT SERVICES IN THE VOLUNTARY SECTOR

# Blackwell: A Case Study in Feminist Administration

Allyson Young Schwartz, MSS
Eve Weiss Gottesman, MSS
Felice Davidson Perlmutter, PhD

Many alternative organizations have focused on the need for social change, both to get at the root of social problems they seek to redress and to address internal problems that may be related to organizational structure. Feminist service agencies, in particular, have a dual focus as they deal with systems change both externally and internally.

While these non-traditional organizations often do not survive, and many of those that do become increasingly traditional in both outlook and structure, some not only have survived but also have remained committed to social change goals and principles. These latter organizations provide valuable insight into a unique constellation of organizational structure and management style.

This paper examines a feminist agency whose mandate is to offer

Ms. Schwartz is Executive Director, Elizabeth Blackwell Health Center for Women, 1124 Walnut Street, Philadelphia, PA 19107. Ms. Gottesman is a member, and a former Chairperson, of the Board of Directors of the Blackwell Center. Dr. Perlmutter is Professor, School of Social Administration, Temple University, Philadelphia, PA 19122.

 

gynecological services to women, and which serves to illustrate an effective alternative organization. The growing literature in this field highlights the radical departure from conventional health services (Stern, 1986) and provides insight into the forces which led to the founding of the Elizabeth Blackwell Health Center for Women, in Philadelphia. This feminist agency has made critical decisions which not only created but have sustained an unconventional management style, while simultaneously protecting its service mandate.

## THEORETICAL ASSUMPTIONS

Feminist administrative theory contains several fundamental assumptions: first, the unique needs of women must be addressed; second, a nonhierarchical, participatory structure is essential; third, the mission of the organization must focus on structural change and not merely the provision of services (Ferguson, 1984). This administrative philosophy serves as an important underpinning for the case study to follow, since it frames the mission of the agency.

Relevant to this discussion is the model of agency development which stems from social systems theory (Perlmutter, 1969) and highlights the centrality of "critical decisions" which agencies make as they grow and change (Selznick, 1957). Attention here is on the evolutionary changes in an organization as it adapts to internal and external requirements while protecting its basic organizational mission and mandate. The discussion focuses on power and decision-making within this alternative agency.

## THE CASE STUDY

### Defining the Mission

The Elizabeth Blackwell Health Center for Women was organized in the summer of 1974 by a group of women who saw a need for non-profit, woman-controlled abortion services. They came together out of a common negative work experience in a commercially financed, physician-owned, for-profit abortion facility. It was thus clear to the founders that the quality of services provided to women is affected by the ownership, philosophy and goals of the organization. These women drew upon the experience of other women around the country who were already involved in self-help clinics and study groups. They sought to apply what they knew of these experiences to their own goals and to their local situation: a large city with an extensive, sophisticated and fairly traditional medical system.

The basic principles defining the mission of the organization reflected those articulated in feminist theory, as follows:

1. Health care is a right; the profit motive in health care can negatively affect quality of care.

2. Women have the right to understand their body functions and control their reproduction.

3. The needs of the consumer should be the utmost consideration in organizing the delivery of health care. . . . Consumers should be active participants in their personal health care and . . . participate in the decision-making activities of the health care system.

4. Health care should . . . emphasize maintenance of health and prevention of disease . . . and take into account physical, mental, social and environmental conditions. It should recognize female reproductive processes as health processes, not sickness.

5. A feminist working environment recognizes the value of every staff member's contribution, guarantees the right of every staff member to participate in decision-making and encourages staff to expand their skills (Blackwell, Statement of Principles, 1975).

Guided by these principles, the founders determined to organize a health center to provide high quality, low cost health services to all kinds of women in a democratic environment which would respect each person and encourage maximal participation by consumers and staff.

During 14 months of planning, the founders made a series of critical decisions which implemented the principles articulated above and which were to govern the organization:

1. The fee-generating services made self-sufficiency and continuity realistic goals. They also allowed a degree of freedom that would have been impossible with complete dependence on grants. Thus, fiscal accountability and fiscal viability were realistic goals from the outset.

2. Start-up funding would not come from an individual or group of individuals who could subsequently, either subtly or overtly, control the organization.

3. The organization would be a non-profit corporation. A Board of Directors, elected by consumers, would be composed of interested individuals (primarily women) who could lend expertise and advice to the Center.

4. Staff would have maximum access to information and decision-making, short of being a collective. This would be accom-

plished, in part, by requiring that one-third of the Board of Directors be staff-elected staff members and that all Board committees include staff representatives (Blackwell, By-Laws, 1976).

5. The organization would seek to limit the traditional disparities of salary and power among staff, although there would be specific and distinct job titles and descriptions, and salaries would vary.

6. The women to be served would be called "consumers" in an effort to enhance their power in their relationships with the service providers at the Center, in contrast to the connotation of powerlessness inherent in the term, "patient." Consumers would be sought from a widely diverse population, since the Center was committed from the outset to serving women of all income levels, ages, racial and ethnic backgrounds and lifestyles, including lesbians as well as heterosexual women, and feminists as well as women who had never identified themselves as feminist.

7. Since an initial goal was to provide services to "women like ourselves," the staff and Board would be representative of the women who were to be served (i.e., race, age, experience and lifestyle) and would provide services they themselves would wish to use.

8. Abortion and contraceptive services would be offered within the context of complete "well-woman" gynecological care.

9. Blackwell would use what was valuable in the traditional health care delivery system, while seeking to expand on that system and to challenge its inequities for both worker and consumer. The philosophies of self-help and participatory health care were incorporated to assure that each woman's experience was validated and recognized and that women sharing with each other would augment the strength and knowledge of all (Blackwell, Statement of Principles, 1975).

### *Program Implementation*

The Center opened in October, 1975, with a staff and Board integrated by race, class, ethnicity, age and education; the Board was somewhat more middle-class, well-educated and professional. Those involved with the Center identified themselves as feminists, but most had not worked in alternative organizations and had little experience in either collectives or self-help groups. The Director was a professional with experience in a consumer-oriented health care delivery system. She was also one of the founders and was strongly committed to the feminist goals and philosophy of the organization.

In 11 years the Center has grown dramatically. In the decade from 1976 to 1986 the annual budget increased from $220,000 to $800,000; services increased from 5,000 to more than 10,000 visits; personnel expanded from eight to 35 full- and part-time staff, from 12 to 40 volunteers and students, and from a 15 to a 21 member Board of Directors.

Funding sources have been fairly consistent, with approximately 80 percent of funds generated through fees for services and 20 percent from foundation grants and private donations. Most private donations come to the Center through Women's Way, a local fundraising coalition of feminist organizations (discussed in a later article in this volume). Except for $2,500 from the Department of Health, Education and Welfare in 1976 for a cancer screening program, there has been no direct government funding of the Center.

The following discussion focuses on power and decision-making at the Blackwell Center, as reflected in: (1) policy and governance, (2) personnel, and (3) services. While these three dimensions are highly interrelated in this agency, for purposes of analysis they will be treated separately.

### *(1) Policy-Making, Planning and Governance*

The issue of power arises in both obvious and subtle ways in all organizations. Some of those involved in alternative organizations are reluctant to acknowledge the reality and legitimacy of authority and power as instrumental in defining relationships and as a functional imperative to accomplishing an organization's movement toward its goals. At Blackwell there has been from the beginning an effort to accept the value of leadership and authority, while, at the same time, recognizing the importance of each staff member's contribution.

Equally important, however, are the checks and balances that limit the accumulation of power. At Blackwell this is done both by assuring accountability of the individual to the whole group (i.e., the entire staff or the Board of Directors) and by devising mechanisms to assure the sharing of power in key decisions. These mechanisms, along with the commitment of the leadership to Blackwell's basic principles, have contributed to the intricate and perhaps unique balance struck between hierarchy and collective structure in the organization. This structure, while complex at times, has enabled the organization to accomplish its goals, to grow and change, while remaining committed to its initial feminist philosophy.

Initially, although each staff member had a specific job description, there was considerable flexibility and job rotation. As the organization matured and the staff grew in number, this diminished; staff members are now less likely to carry responsibilities or perform tasks unrelated to their own jobs. Nonetheless, significant time and energy are devoted to including all staff in problem-solving and decision-making. For example, all staff have the opportunity to serve on Board committees and attend Board meetings.

Considerable attention is given to creating mechanisms by which all levels of staff can respond to issues which affect the organization. For example, the administrative staff work to frame questions so that all staff can focus on an issue, consider options, voice opinions and arrive at agreement on direction. However, interest in and ability to share decision-making authority must be worked at by all staff. Most new staff have to "unlearn" attitudes of powerlessness inherent in most traditional workplaces and have to be reminded of the mechanisms provided for direct involvement in decision-making. Staff's willingness to speak openly about policy issues and to attempt to consider the larger impact on the organization, as well as their own positions on an issue, is one of the positive aspects of their shared commitment to relating to each other in a more collective way. But this is also a difficult process and one which requires an active and conscious commitment.

This process is also used to modify programs and plan new ones. Ideas for new programs are still generated informally by staff during the year, or by the Board in its annual long-range planning process, in which goals and objectives for the year are delineated in detail. This process pushes the Center to plan concretely for the following year and to consider goals for a number of years ahead. The Birth Center, for example, involved several years of consideration and planning before implementation was possible. There is increasing pressure from the Board for a five-year plan for the Center, and a permanent planning committee has been formed. While this will formalize the planning process, it is hoped that it will not diminish Blackwell's flexibility and responsiveness to community needs but, rather, enhance its ability to meet those needs.

## *(2) Personnel*

Staff relationships at Blackwell reflect not only the principles articulated earlier, but also the informality which is possible in a small agency. From the inception of the agency until recently, staff reported to the Executive Director or the Assistant Director and rejected additional levels of hierarchy.

Over time the agency grew more complex by adding staff, diversifying services and delineating staff roles more precisely. To accommodate this growth, some staff began to play supervisory roles with students, volunteers and other staff. This informal supervision led to the need to clarify responsibilities and identify appropriate levels of supervision. The Board and staff agreed to recognize and legitimize certain lines of accountability, which were already operational. In this process roles were refined and other lines of accountability were also clarified. These refinements, however, have not changed the basic structure, in which all staff have access to information and decision-making. Staff still relate to each other as peers, despite differences in salaries, job titles and responsibilities.

Other key areas of decision-making include hiring and firing, staff evaluations and salary. These areas most severely challenge staff's ability to see beyond their own needs and feelings to that which might be best for the organization.

Hiring and firing of all staff, except the Executive Director, is the responsibility of a staff committee whose membership is rotated among all staff on a quarterly basis. This committee also decides on the salaries to be paid to new staff, within ranges set by a Board committee. The Executive Director is hired by the Board of Directors, and, since staff members serve on the Board, staff are thus also involved in this process. This illustrates the blend of traditional (the Board hiring the Executive Director and setting salary ranges) and alternative (staff hiring each other) organizational models.

With regard to evaluations, all staff members are evaluated annually by all others. These written performance evaluations are reviewed with the staff person and the Executive and Assistant Directors. An unsatisfactory evaluation, or performance poor enough to question continuation of the employee, is brought before the staff committee for formal review and determination. Staff members have been put on probation or have been fired by this committee, in a process both lengthy and, at times, painful.

Salary decisions, although related to issues of power and authority, are also viewed vis-à-vis Blackwell's organizing principles, which attempt to deal with problems of distributive justice. The matter of salary disparity has become a more prominent issue as the organization has grown and become more professionalized. At the outset, salaries were disparate but not dramatically so. Several factors have led to increasing disparity in salaries: (1) the longevity of some staff, particularly at the upper ranges, (2) changes in job descriptions, and (3) the addition of staff with advanced professional training.

One means to deal with disparities is the mechanism for salary increases developed by the Board and staff in 1982. Before this time there were either no increases or an across-the-board amount. After much discussion, it was decided that a staff member would receive a set increase on the anniversary date of her employment, the amount ($300 to $500) based on the number of years employed at the Center. In addition, the Board would grant an annual cost-of-living increase, which in odd years would be a percentage of the individual's salary and in even years a percentage of the median salary. In this way the disparity issue would be addressed at least in part. While there is some grumbling in the even years, most of the staff are committed to this concept. In fact, the issue has surfaced only when a major revision in ranges or salaries is discussed and is not an ongoing problem.

### *(3) Services*

The Blackwell Center offers a wide range of women's health care services and programs. From the outset it has offered well-woman gynecological care, including contraception, pregnancy testing and options counseling, abortion services, health education (e.g., workshops on self-help and consumer rights and presentations on a variety of health issues). In addition, the Center has always provided gynecological care for women past childbearing age and for others not concerned about contraception, as well as for those interested in various reproductive options.

At present, the Center's services include full maternity care, with an out-of-hospital birth center staffed by certified nurse-midwives, early second trimester abortions, insemination for fertile women, dispensing the cervical cap (a barrier method contraceptive) as part of an FDA testing program, and educational programs on menopause, hysterectomy, fertility awareness, nutrition, and childbearing options.

The Center continues to advocate for women's rights—politically, for access to health care, and for control over their reproductive decisions.

Over the years, new services have been added both in response to consumer interest and based on staff and Board perceptions of needs in the community and appropriate directions for Blackwell. However, there never has been a clear, defined means by which these perceptions were to be articulated and responses agreed upon by staff and Board. Trial and error has been the method of expediency, if not choice.

One example of the way the system has worked is demonstrated by the addition of the controversial artificial insemination service in 1982. The Director and some staff had become aware that two other women's health centers in the Northeastern United States were offering artificial insemination in their communities. In response to some local interest, discussion was initiated at staff meetings. This was further encouraged by some interest on the Board in initiating such a service for fertile women who were unable to conceive for social reasons (i.e., primarily lesbians or single heterosexual women). The idea was approved by the Board, and planning proceeded.

The intention to offer the insemination service was announced informally by the Director in the monthly newsletter for Center volunteers. The Director felt secure that the staff had the necessary technical expertise to handle an insemination service competently and became committed to the idea of offering it to fill a perceived service need in the community. The staff, however, unexpectedly raised serious concerns about their own expertise in this area and about the decision to offer the service at that time. Their ambivalence may be reflective of the dichotomy identified by Clarke (1956), in which he suggests that new, risk-taking programs often reflect "precarious" values, as opposed to more readily acceptable programs, which are based on "secure" values.

In response to these concerns, two Board members offered to lead a discussion on the topic and focused on the unarticulated issues underlying the concern about the insemination service. Some of the staff's concern had to do with the expectation that they, who had been trained not to be judgmental about women's reproductive decisions, might have to make judgments about who should or should not become a mother. The discussions were helpful and resulted in a clear affirmation of the staff's feelings about helping women to carry out their reproductive options. Assurances were made regarding the importance of obtaining relevant medical and legal advice and identifying certain contraindications, such as alcoholism or drug addiction. Staff members committed themselves to learning what was necessary to offer a high quality service, and it turned out to be a positive learning experience for the entire organization.

The experience confirmed the importance of obtaining staff consensus, based on adequate information and involvement, before initiating a new service or program. Subsequently, the expansion of services in other areas, such as later abortion procedures, and gynecology services for physically disabled and mentally retarded women, were introduced only after a solid foundation of support was laid with both staff and Board.

## *SUMMARY AND IMPLICATIONS*

Blackwell is an agency which has successfully applied its principles and philosophy to an expanding service, growing staff and changing times. It remains committed to its original goals but has been willing to modify the mechanisms used to achieve them. It continues to take what is valuable from more traditional systems and channel it into innovative ways of providing services and managing an organization. This requires a vision of what the agency should be, a consistent commitment to the organizational goals, and a willingness to look at itself.

The Center has had the good fortune to be in touch with a network of feminist health providers in other areas of the country with whom to discuss ideas and issues, as well as with a group of other feminist organizations in the City which offer interaction and support. Both networks have reduced isolation and helped assure that the Center stays in tune with the larger feminist movement and with other alternative service agencies.

During its existence, the Center's definition of its goals and philosophy has changed little. The mechanisms devised to achieve the goals are basically intact. However, over the years modifications have been made to accommodate growth and change. Some of these can be pinpointed as to time and place, but most have been slow and evolutionary. The Board, the leadership and the staff have responded to needs for change with creativity and continued commitment to the mission of the organization.

The mechanisms developed and the decisions made by this agency are worthy of attention by other non-profit service organizations and may be useful in addressing issues related to participatory management, empowerment, effectiveness and commitment to purpose – all issues addressed directly or indirectly by such organizations.

## REFERENCES

By-Laws of the Elizabeth Blackwell Health Center for Women, Philadelphia, 1976.

Clark, B.R. Organizational adaptation and precarious values. *American Sociological Review*, 1956, *21*, 327-336.

Ferguson, K.E. *The feminist case against bureaucracy*. Philadelphia: Temple University Press, 1984.

Perlmutter, F.D. A theoretical model of social agency development. *Social Casework*, 1969, *50*, 467-473.

Selznick, P. *Leadership in administration*. New York: Harper & Row, 1957.

Statement of Principles of the Elizabeth Blackwell Health Center for Women, Philadelphia, 1975.

Stern, P.N. *Women, health and culture*. Washington, DC: Hemisphere Publishing Corporation, 1986.

# Shanti: An Alternative Response to the AIDS Crisis

Nancy R. Hooyman, PhD
Karen I. Fredriksen, MSW
Barbara Perlmutter, MSW

Social and health service professionals' general insensitivity to and lack of information about issues faced by gays and lesbians have long been problematic (Messing, Schoenberg, & Stephens, 1984; Dulaney & Kelly, 1982). Such insensitivity and misinformation have been highlighted by the helping professions' inadequate response to the specific psychosocial needs of people with AIDS (acquired immune deficiency syndrome), the majority of whom thus far are gay men and intravenous drug abusers (Lopez & Getzel, 1984). The occurrence of AIDS has engendered widespread anxiety in the public mind, diverting attention from the enormous problems facing people with AIDS. Such anxiety undoubtedly underlies instances where people with AIDS have been socially isolated, dismissed from their jobs, evicted from their homes, received inadequate health care, or even been denied social and health services (NASW, 1984; Cecchi, 1986). Health and social service professionals have gradually begun to become more aware of the needs of people with AIDS. Nevertheless, both those with AIDS, as well as populations at high risk of contracting AIDS, often still face social ostracism and direct abuse of their rights as citizens (Lopez & Getzel, 1984).

---

Dr. Hooyman is Dean, School of Social Work, University of Washington, Seattle, WA 98195. Ms. Fredriksen is Senior Care Coordinator, Ballard Community Hospital, P.O. Box C70707, Seattle, WA 98107. Ms. Perlmutter is Outpatient Therapist, Seattle Mental Health Institute, 1600 E. Olive Street, Seattle, WA 98122. Ms. Fredriksen and Ms. Perlmutter were among the founders of Shanti.

 

Although AIDS was first recognized as a perplexing and tragic medical phenomenon, the intrinsic psychosocial dimensions of AIDS – the shattering emotional reactions of those who have the illness, those who are at risk and those who are a family member, friend or lover of a person with AIDS – must also be attended to by health and social service professionals. Because of the prognosis associated with AIDS, the initial diagnosis, in and of itself, can be emotionally devastating. Typical psychological responses that accompany the diagnosis include fears of death and the dying process; guilt, isolation and stigmatization, confusion and concern over options for medical treatment; and an overriding sense of despair, helplessness, social rejection and the loss of esteem typically associated with terminal illness and, often for gay men, the exposure of sexual orientation. Because the fear of AIDS tends to be compounded by homophobia (an irrational fear of homosexuals), persons with AIDS may also find themselves without the support of families, friends, and co-workers.

Traditional health and social service systems, preoccupied with the provision of medical care, reimbursement constraints, and cost-containment, may be unable to respond adequately to the "roller coaster" ride of emotional reactions experienced by persons with AIDS (Lopez & Getzel, 1984). For example, interviews with people with AIDS have shown that although their medical needs were generally addressed adequately, their psychological needs were not given sufficient attention (Morin, Charles, & Malyon, 1984). Human service professionals who work with persons with AIDS are caught in a powerful dilemma: They need to support the person in overcoming immediate crises through problem-solving and the provision of concrete services while simultaneously enabling the person to explore the wide range of feelings associated with his/her remaining life, dying process and death. A crisis intervention model of social work practice, for example, fails to capture the special qualities of intervention required with people with AIDS (Golan, 1978).

In an effort to respond to this dual dilemma, Shanti, a Seattle-based alternative agency, focuses on meeting the emotional needs of persons with life-threatening illnesses and those grieving another's death. Although Shanti was formed to address psychosocial needs associated with all types of life-threatening illnesses, it now primarily serves people with AIDS or AIDS-related conditions, and those grieving the loss of a person from AIDS. In addition to providing emotional support to individuals, Shanti serves the larger community through public speaking and education, information and referral, and providing training and technical assistance to community organizations.

This article (1) reviews Shanti's mission and objectives and how these have changed over time in response to the growing AIDS crisis; (2) describes the decision-making structure that has evolved from these objectives to meet the changing needs of clients and volunteers; (3) identifies the major strengths and limitations of this structure for serving the unique needs of people with AIDS and other life-threatening illnesses; and (4) suggests implications for those presently engaged in designing and delivering services for persons with AIDS. One of the more striking characteristics of Shanti is how its objectives, the clients served, and the characteristics of volunteers have shifted over a relatively short time period in response to the rapidly changing social context created by the growing AIDS epidemic. These rapid internal and external changes, which have placed extraordinary demands on people's energies, are also discussed.

## *LITERATURE REVIEW*

The development of Shanti as an alternative service is consistent with Grossman and Morgenbesser's (1980) definition of alternative agencies which view themselves as departing significantly in terms of goals, modes of operation, philosophy, and structure from the traditional social service network. According to Grossman and Morgenbesser, the founders of alternative organizations are usually motivated by the desire to meet the needs of an unserved, underserved or inappropriately served group; the initial funding is outside of traditional agency, community or governmental sources; staff may have some professional training, but their primary characteristic is direct identification with the client group to be served. Collaborative, equalitarian structures are emphasized. Similarly, Rothschild-Whitt (1979) characterized alternative organizations by their small size, economic marginality, internal support base, diffusion of knowledge for task performance among staff positions, and mutual and self-criticism of the members or volunteers. According to Kanter and Zurcher (1973), alternative organizations value small size for allowing more interaction and attention to individual needs. Organizational stability is less important than the potential for growth and change, with the process as product. The concept of wholeness translates into efforts to integrate personal and professional aspects of member's lives, to assert the importance of relationships, and to value the person as a whole.

According to Parsons and Hodne (1982), founders of alternative organizations choose to develop an alternative services structure rather than directly challenging and trying to change the larger social and health care system. In the process of establishing an alternative structure, founders must continually assess who they want to reach, the resources available, and whether their strategy of a separate agency is politically feasible. Careful assessment of these questions is necessary both for the immediate objectives of providing direct services and the long-term objectives of organizational growth.

Although research on alternative organizations is limited compared to that on traditional bureaucracies, there appear to be characteristic dilemmas that arise in the development of alternative service agencies. These dilemmas contrast with the life-cycle stages of self-interest, professionalism, and social interest typical of traditional social agencies (Perlmutter, 1969). One dilemma faced by most alternative organizations is achieving a balance between process and product (Crow, 1978; Riddle, 1978). For example, in the development of alternative health services for women, Parsons and Hodne (1982) noted the failure of one organization to delegate responsibility and share ownership of the project with all workers, while another rotated jobs too quickly. In one health clinic, insufficient attention was paid to reaching consensus, while in another, the time spent on processing group decisions inhibited the ability to carry out tasks essential to the clinic's operation. Although the original members of alternative organizations generally share a value commitment to the importance of process, time pressures, increased size, or the demands of outside funders may result in a move toward greater task specialization in an effort to "get the job done." When knowledge needed to perform the organization's tasks becomes unevenly distributed, the alternative structure tends to be undermined, pushing it in the direction of power inequities (Rothschild-Whitt, 1979). Yet it is unlikely that all members will be equally skilled and interested in performing all administrative and direct service tasks, a factor that over time works against shared responsibilities.

Staff turnover generally has a negative impact on the maintenance of alternative structures. New staff may not share the founder's commitment to collective goals and structure, and therefore may not value diffusion of knowledge among staff nor more informal processes of decision-making. Rapid changes in staff composition may also disrupt the personal relationships that are conducive to collective decision-making. Without such strong personal ties and shared commitment to the collective structure, new staff may be more comfortable with specialization and formal structure than were the founders (Morgenbesser et al., 1981).

External funding, more than any other factor, generally alters the structure of alternative organizations (Morgenbesser et al., 1981). This is because external funding often carries other requirements, such as a board of directors, a designated division of labor, or changes in the types of clients served. When funding is readily available, the temptation to accept such funding, despite the "strings" attached, becomes strong. In addition, linkages to traditional agencies through in-service education, referral networks, and community boards can intensify the pressure to accept outside resources. According to Rothschild-Whitt (1979), organizational dependence on an external base of support tends to increase the likelihood of goal displacement and to decrease the level of internal participation by members, staff, or clients. Internal participation declines largely because as staff devote time to writing grant proposals and cultivating funding agencies, they simply have less time to attend to volunteers and clients.

As the following case study illustrates, Shanti has faced similar dilemmas in its development: conflicts between process and product, staff burnout from administrative responsibilities to which they were less committed than to direct service tasks, resultant staff turnover, and increasing pressures from the larger environment as the AIDS epidemic has escalated and the funding for services to people with AIDS has grown.

## *ORIGINS OF SHANTI*

The Seattle-based Shanti was started in 1983 by four volunteers, three women and one man, each cognizant of the need for such a service from their own personal experiences of loss. They were trained by the fifteen-year-old Shanti Project in San Francisco. Although not formally related, Shanti Project served as a model for the organizers of Shanti in Seattle. In 1983, social and health professionals were just becoming aware of the AIDS epidemic. Even though the founders defined Shanti as serving the full spectrum of those who were dying or grieving, they also recognized the lack of support services for those with AIDS or AIDS-related illnesses. The founders of Shanti therefore viewed themselves as developing an alternative structure to meet a growing and critical need in the community. Similar to the health clinics studied by Parsons and Hodne (1982), the founders deliberately chose to develop separate services to meet the growing need rather than to try to change existing agencies, such as hospice, which did not share their commitment to AIDS and gay-sensitivity, nor Shanti's other goals and objectives.

### *Mission and Objectives*

Shanti, a volunteer psychosocial support organization, serves individuals facing a life-threatening illness or grieving the loss of a loved one. A primary objective of Shanti is to provide free, confidential emotional support to individuals, both from the gay/lesbian community and from the community at large. Equally important is a focus on the personal growth, development, and support of volunteers. Shanti's philosophy emphasizes volunteers' learning to care for themselves in the process of caring for others.

In meeting these objectives, Shanti explicitly chose to be different from traditional services in a number of ways. Although hospice programs exist in local hospitals and home care agencies, eligibility for their volunteer services tends to be linked to receiving professionally provided skilled nursing services, which are expensive, or to those who are Medicare or insurance-eligible. Shanti provides services without charge regardless of a person's income, age, sex, race, religion, marital status or sexual preference. Social-emotional needs are emphasized rather than primarily providing respite care or assisting with the practical activities of daily living and medical concerns. Clients are served during all phases of a life-threatening illness, in contrast to hospice services which are generally limited to those in their last few months of life. Shanti also differs from most hospice-related agencies in its commitment to serving the dying person's family and loved ones as primary clients with or without the dying person's involvement. By defining family to include non-related persons, Shanti reaches those who might not be recognized and supported by more traditional agencies. At the most basic level, Shanti's founders did not want to create another hospice; instead they intended to provide those facing a life-threatening illness and their loved ones, including gays, lesbians and people with AIDS, with a deliberately structured alternative that would primarily address their emotional needs. The impetus for Shanti is thus similar to that of most alternative organizations: to meet the needs of an unserved, underserved, or inappropriately served group and to work with others who share similar philosophical beliefs and values (Grossman & Morgenbesser, 1980).

### *Decision-Making Structure*

An emphasis on collective and equalitarian structure tends to be part of the shared beliefs and values. During Shanti's first two years, the four founders were largely responsible for planning and administering the organization—setting policy; program development; screening, training, and supervising volunteers; providing information and referral services; day-to-day administration, public relations, and marketing; and working with other service organizations. Simultaneously, all staff provided clinical services. For the founders, Shanti was a way of life, a full-time commitment, for which they received no financial compensation.

Although Shanti has designated staff who coordinate services, there are no paid staff. All persons, including staff, volunteer to work with Shanti. Volunteers, including the staff coordinators, are therefore both service providers and policy-makers. The underlying philosophy that all volunteers should have the opportunity to learn all tasks was reflected in the low level of specialization at this stage of organizational development. As a result, personal development of volunteers was often emphasized at the expense of long-range organizational development. In other words, priority was placed upon involving volunteers in both service and administrative responsibilities, rather than assigning tasks according to individuals' abilities or preferences.

Organizational and administrative decisions were made by consensus. If consensus could not be reached, policies were not changed. This emphasis on consensus reflects the founders' commitment to collaboration and shared decision-making. Frequent feedback from volunteers and clients was also encouraged by staff. For example, staff meetings were open to all volunteers. Clients were systematically contacted for their feedback approximately six to eight weeks after being matched with a Shanti volunteer. These efforts at generating feedback and shared decision-making have generally resulted in decisions that reflected the needs of all three constituencies – clients, volunteers, and staff.

When consensus could not be reached, staff and volunteers agreed upon the following principles for resolving conflicts. Each person was committed to giving and receiving feedback and to assuming responsibility for resolving issues, whether or not he or she was personally involved in the issue. As much time as needed was taken to deal with the conflict. If the conflict was not resolved, an outside person was brought in to assist in problem-resolution.

Since its founding, Shanti's structure has changed as a result of the growing numbers of new staff and volunteers. This growth resulted primarily from the escalating AIDS epidemic and with it, both the demand for Shanti to provide services to more people with AIDS and the increased need to obtain outside funding. The newcomers who replaced the original staff were frequently pressured by the need to respond to the growing community problem of AIDS. In addition, Shanti was called upon to participate in intra-agency planning meetings and task forces regarding the development of AIDS services – external demands that vied for the limited amount of time and energy available for responding to intra-agency needs.

Along with the growing number of volunteers and clients served, work demands intensified, new staff were added, and the level of specialization increased. Consistent with the effects of staff turnover and increased size noted by Morgenbesser et al. (1981), a departure from the original staff-directed structure emerged. Five task-oriented committees were established. These committees, composed of volunteers, are: office support, public relations, volunteer and client services, fund-raising, and long-range planning. All committees include a staff person, who serves as coordinator and sits on a committee of coordinators. This coordinating committee (e.g., the staff) receives input from each of the five committees, providing the overall structure for decision-making and policy direction. All committees operate according to a consensus model of decision-making. Major decisions are brought before the entire membership for feedback and occasionally for a vote. However, the current organization is also planning to implement a board composed of volunteers, clients, and outside representatives, a move which appears to be a shift away from an emphasis upon shared decision-making solely by staff and volunteers.

### *The Central Role of Volunteers*

The extent to which Shanti relies upon volunteers and emphasizes their emotional growth as part of its overall mission and objectives also differentiates it from other agencies. As noted above, all persons volunteer to work with Shanti. Shanti has demonstrated major strengths in the area of providing its volunteers with a wide range of opportunities for personal and professional development as service providers, administrators, policy-makers, and trainers.

Shanti has also been effective in recruiting a diverse pool of volunteers. As the AIDS epidemic has escalated, and with it Shanti's response, the range of individuals who make the service commitment to Shanti reflect the growing recognition of AIDS as a community concern, not only a gay concern. Volunteers of both sexes, diverse ages, lifestyles, educational levels and backgrounds are actively involved in all phases of the organization. Such a varied group of volunteers has permitted a valuable exchange of information and experiences among volunteers, as well as assisted in meeting the individual needs of each client.

The process of volunteering, which in itself builds support for volunteers, begins with the completion of an in-depth application, followed by a careful personal screening interview. These measures are intended to serve both the potential volunteer and the trainers in determining the suitability of volunteering at Shanti. If both parties agree, the next step is participation in the 40-hour intensive training. This is both experiential and educational, and covers two consecutive weekends. Throughout the training, support and feedback are provided to volunteers. If the trainee successfully completes the training, an invitation to join Shanti is extended. At that time, volunteers are asked to commit to one year of service and to volunteer a minimum of five hours a week; this encompasses working with clients, attending a weekly supervision and support group, and participating in optional committee work. The two-hour supervision and support group is the primary mechanism of support and is specifically structured to promote emotional growth and prevent burnout by providing volunteers with opportunities to process the feelings which arise in relation to their work with clients. It is also the place where volunteers receive feedback about their own development and their work with clients.

Another method that supports the volunteers' growth is the encouragement to participate in subsequent volunteer training sessions, to act as support/supervision group co-leaders, and to assume new administrative and organizational tasks both within Shanti and within the larger social service community. Thus, the volunteer chooses whether to develop administrative skills while acquiring peer counseling skills.

### *Preventing Burnout*

The risk of burnout exists in most service work. When working with people with AIDS, the risk of burnout is even greater, largely because of working primarily with young people for whom death is now inevitable, the debilitating physical and mental progression of the disease, and the societal isolation and rejection surrounding people with AIDS. Many volunteers have chosen to work with Shanti because of their own experiences with grief and, increasingly, with AIDS. Many of them have lost a friend or loved one to AIDS. Many of them have lost a friend or loved one to AIDS. A Shanti volunteer was recently diagnosed with Kaposi's Sarcoma, one of AIDS' lethal opportunistic illnesses. Volunteers are being increasingly called upon to support each other as AIDS claims the lives of clients, friends, and co-workers.

Although the sensitivity and skill of volunteers are undoubtedly enhanced by such experiences, their emotional vulnerability may be heightened. Regardless of past experiences, the work performed by volunteers is extremely demanding emotionally. There is often a waiting list of clients needing services. Given these pressures, volunteers could easily slip into a "helper" role, where there is always more to do and one has never done enough.

Shanti staff have deliberately aimed to minimize burnout by requiring that volunteers participate in training, support groups, and retreats. A strong support system is created by frequent telephoning, "checking in," and socializing among volunteers. The training program and support groups emphasize taking care of oneself, not solely caretaking others. Volunteers focus on cultivating self-forgiveness and self-acceptance as a way to acknowledge their own needs and recognize their own limits. The hope of developing caring and compassion for themselves in order to provide caring and compassionate service to others is a cornerstone of Shanti's philosophy. Shanti staff also believe that burnout occurs when people do not allow themselves to face their own emotions. Providing opportunities for volunteers to confront their own feelings is viewed as essential to renewing their energy in order to provide sustained support to dying and grieving individuals. In addition, volunteers are deliberately affirmed for their ability to have responded to 150 persons who would otherwise have been inadequately served in the community during the past three years. Shanti therefore represents a model of self-caretaking as well as for providing services to the dying and grieving.

However, burnout from administrative tasks tends to be higher than from the emotionally demanding work with clients. As policy-makers, administrators, and direct service workers, volunteers are involved in all aspects of administering the organization. Yet most volunteers choose to be involved in Shanti because of the chance to work directly with clients and to confront their own issues of loss, not because of organizational opportunities. As Shanti has grown, volunteers increasingly find themselves devoting more time to administrative and organizational development tasks. These time demands can be especially constraining for the majority of volunteers who are employed full-time, many of them in other service capacities.

### *Funding Base*

Funding has always been a critical issue for Shanti. The reliance on volunteers as both policy-makers and direct service providers stems largely from an ideological position. Another primary force behind the use of volunteers is a more practical one – the limited funding available for alternative services, such as Shanti. To compound this situation, most persons with AIDS are minorities, historically disfavored by mainstream American society. The funds available for AIDS services were, until recently, extremely limited. Even as the demand for AIDS services increased and partial funding became available, resources for social services for persons with AIDS have had lower priority than research, prevention, and education. Shanti has lacked the volunteer resources to devote full-time to fund-raising efforts, and for the first 2 1/2 years relied primarily upon donations and small-scale fund-raising efforts. Priority was initially placed on the type and quality of services which were provided rather than on rapid growth or obtaining external funding for long-range development. However, with the increased availability of funds for direct services to persons with AIDS, current Shanti staff has placed priority on obtaining external funding. What is unknown is the extent that these fund-raising efforts will, over time, result in less attention to the personal development needs of volunteers (Rothschild-Whitt, 1979).

Shanti recently received operating expenses and office space from the local AIDS fund-raising organization. This physical move from one of the founder's homes to their office in itself is a reflection of the staff's increased priority on serving people with AIDS. Having set this priority, staff are faced with the reality that resources for people with AIDS are gradually increasing, but that little funding exists for services to those who are dying and grieving as a result of other types of illnesses. As another step in the process of obtaining funding, Shanti is planning on establishing a board of directors, thereby moving away from having only staff and volunteers as policy-makers. Shanti has also been included in recent grant-writing efforts for services to people with AIDS, which, if funded, will create paid positions for a full-time volunteer coordinator and part-time clerical support. If granted, Shanti would be obligated to serve more people than previously, as well as to increase the number of volunteers dramatically—all changes which may alter Shanti's alternative structure.

### *Implications*

In sum, Shanti has undergone significant changes since its inception. During its development, it has faced a dilemma common to most alternative organizations: how to achieve a balance between process and task performance (Crow, 1978). Shanti has also experienced the additional tension of how to provide sufficient time for conflict resolution and the personal growth of volunteers while needing to devote tremendous energies to organizational demands.

Although reliance on highly committed volunteers is central to Shanti as an alternative service agency and, in fact, has been one of its major strengths, it has also presented organizational problems. Due to volunteer burnout from administrative and organizational demands, staff turnover has been fairly high. Morgenbesser et al. (1981) found that staff and volunteers who join an alternative organization after its creation are often less involved in viewing the agency as a primary reference group and are less uncomfortable with specialization and formal structure. Rapid changes in staff composition can also disrupt the personal relationships that seem to facilitate collective management. As original Shanti staff have been replaced by newcomers, increased priority has been placed on serving people with AIDS, expanding in size, establishing a board, and obtaining outside funding.

In addition, the administrative tasks that have consumed considerable staff time have tended to be those required for daily operation. As a result, issues of long-range planning, program development and fund-raising have been inadequately addressed. Also compounding this situation has been the changing nature of the organization's larger social context: the growing AIDS epidemic, the lack of services to meet such needs, and the increased availability of external funds for services to people with AIDS, all of which have resulted in increasing service specialization. Although Shanti continues to maintain a structure that contrasts with more hierarchical agencies, factors such as these make it vulnerable to goal displacement and movement toward a more traditional structure (Rothschild-Whitt, 1979; Morgenbesser et al., 1981; Parsons & Hodne, 1982).

These findings raise several implications for other alternative organizations. Early in Shanti's development, it would have been useful to have devoted additional time to defining collective goals; for example, to what extent should Shanti serve only persons with AIDS and their families, or the larger population of individuals who are dying or grieving? The periodic reevaluation of such goals and appropriate strategies for meeting them would also have been helpful.

Through both Shanti's philosophy and integrated service elements, a high priority has been to prevent burnout from performance of direct service tasks. The potential for burnout from administrative tasks, however, has not been as clearly recognized nor addressed. More efforts to meet the administrators' needs, through frequent staff retreats and other structured support activities, might have served to reduce staff burnout and turnover. Such structures might also have served to clarify and resolve individual differences among staff.

An additional problem facing Shanti throughout its development has been that major organizational needs, such as long-range planning, program development and fund-raising, have not been met adequately, due largely to the volunteers' time constraints and areas of interest. This problem might have been reduced if more volunteers with administrative interest and skills had been specifically recruited to participate in Shanti. Another option would have been to recognize the necessity of delegating responsibility for specialized tasks without sacrificing the benefits of exchanging skills and information through some job rotation (Parsons & Hodne, 1982). A more traditional approach might have been to seek funds in order to hire a staff person to assist with ongoing fund-raising and long-range development, or to utilize an outside consultant specializing in organizational development. Although options such as these might have reduced administrative burnout and met long-range organizational goals—and may actually become a reality as Shanti increases in size and staff—the extent to which they jeopardize Shanti's alternative structure is as yet unknown.

## REFERENCES


Cecchi, R. Living with AIDS: When the system fails. *American Journal of Nursing*, 1986, *86*(1), 45-47.

Crow, G. The process/product split. *Quest*, 1978, *4*(4), 15-23.

Dulaney, D., & Kelly, J. Improving services to gay and lesbian clients. *Journal of Social Work*, 1982, *27*(2), 178-183.

Furstenberg, A., & Olson, M.M. Social Work and AIDS. *Social Work in Health Care*, 1984, *9*(4), 45-60.

Golan, N. *Treatment in crisis situations*. New York: Free Press, 1978.

Grossman, B., & Morgenbesser, M. Alternative social service settings: Opportunities for social work education. *Journal of Humanics*, 1980, *8*, 59-76.

Kanter, R.M., & Zurcher, L. Concluding statement: Evaluating alternatives and alternative valuing. *The Journal of Applied Behavioral Science*, 1973, *9*(2/3), 381-397.

Lopez, D., & Getzel, G. Helping gay AIDS patients in crisis. *Social Casework*, 1984, *65*(7), 387-394.

Messing, A., Schoenberg, R., & Stephens, R. Confronting homophobia in health care settings: Guidelines for social work practice. Special issue on homosexuality and social work. *Journal of Social Work and Human Sexuality*, 1984, *2*(2/3), 65-74.

Morgenbesser, M., et al. The evolution of three alternative social service agencies. *Catalyst*, 1981, *11*, 71-83.

Morin, S., et al. The psychological impact of AIDS on gay men. *American Psychologist*, 1984, *39*(11), 1288-1293.

National Association of Social Workers. *Acquired immune deficiency syndrome, public social policy statement*. Silver Spring, MD: NASW, September, 1984.

Parsons, P., & Hodne, C. A collective experiment in women's health. *Science for the People*, July/August 1982, 9-13.

Perlmutter, F.D. A theoretical model for social agency development. *Social Casework*, October 1969, *50*(8), 467-473.

Riddle, D. Integrating process and product. *Quest*, 1978, *4*(4), 15-23.

Rothschild-Whitt, J. Conditions for democracy: Making participatory organizations work. In J. Case & R. Taylor (Eds.), *Co-ops, communes and collectives*. New York: Pantheon Books, 1979.

# The Hospice in Transition: Organizational and Administrative Perspectives

Burton Gummer, PhD

The past two decades have seen the growth of a group of human service organizations known as "alternative institutions" (Miller & Phillip, 1983). In addition to hospices, the subject of the present discussion, alternative service agencies now work in the areas of drug and alcohol abuse, physical and mental disability, deinstitutionalized populations, the homeless, battered wives, and gay men and women. The word "alternative" refers both to the kind of service offered and to the organizational structures for providing them, both of which differ from traditional social service organizations.

While these organizations often began as self-help groups or extensions of social and political movements with an anti-establishment ideology, many, like the hospice, have been in operation long enough, and have attracted sufficiently stable sources of clients and funds, to be on the threshold of becoming part of the establishment—that is, of becoming like the bureaucratic service organizations to which they were initially an alternative. The present paper examines one such organization, the hospice, from the perspective of the organizational and administrative alternatives that have developed in them, and what might be done to preserve them as they move from informal associations of like-minded and committed individuals to bureaucratically-organized and professionally-staffed service organizations.

Ours has been called a "bureaucratic society" because of the

---

Dr. Gummer is Associate Professor, School of Social Welfare, Rockefeller College of Public Affairs & Policy, State University of New York at Albany, Albany, NY 12222. This article is a revised version of a paper presented at the Annual Meeting of the New York State Hospice Association, Syracuse, NY, April 15, 1985.

 

amount of work conducted within bureaucratic organizations. The complex, hierarchical organization has become the standard way for organizing tasks as varied as manufacturing silicon chips, making motion pictures, playing baseball, or tending to the sick and dying. The prevalence of this organizational form is due, in great part, to its capacity to produce goods and services efficiently and speedily. From this perspective, bureaucratic organizations have been a boon to humankind by helping to make more goods and services available to more people. One has only to consider the impact of Henry Ford's bureaucratically arranged assembly line on America and the world as the automobile went from being a plaything of the rich to an important part of acceptable standards of living for ordinary people everywhere.

As the bureaucratic organization replaced the family and the local community as the preferred way for doing work, it moved from being just another alternative work arrangement to the status of a social institution. As a result, the hierarchical organization is no longer seen as *a* way of performing work—it is, with few exceptions, *the* way. As with other social institutions, moreover, the bureaucratic organization is the standard against which other structures for organizing work are evaluated. Seeley (1957) suggests that evaluations of alternatives to a central institution have a definite form: An alternative can be a *poor copy* of the ideal form, a *complementary system*, the *best defense* the central institution can have against other alternatives, or a *contradiction* of the central institution.

A hospice, for example, can be evaluated in terms of how similar or different it is from nursing homes and extended care facilities; that is, how good a "copy" it is. Alternatively, it can be seen as part of a chronic care system whose role is to complement other facilities, or a "best defense" whose function is to relieve some of the fiscal pressures on the health system by providing a less expensive form of care. Finally, it can be viewed as an alternative service organized around principles and practices different from those that shape traditional care facilities.

These notions about the evolution of complex organizations provide a framework for examining the organizational and administrative issues facing hospices in the United States, and some possible strategies for addressing them. In particular, they enable us to identify ways in which hospices can avoid becoming "poor copies" of the established approaches to caring for the dying, particularly since dissatisfaction with many of those practices was a factor in the hospice's creation.

## *THE GROWTH OF ORGANIZATIONS: ALTERNATIVE PATHS*

One view of organizational development holds that there are two ways in which organizational structures arise (Meyer et al., 1981). In the first, technological innovations foster the development of bureaucratic structures to coordinate technical work efficiently. In the second, social processes emerge that define certain rules and programs, and the organizations that incorporate these programs and conform to these rules, as rational and legitimate. The emergence of the factory reflects the first way, while the development of the human service organization reflects the second.

While the hospice exists in an environment with a high rate of technological innovation, the impetus for its development came mainly from changes in attitudes towards illness and death. The 1960s have been referred to as the decade of the "citizen participation revolution" as people demanded to be involved in decisions affecting their lives. The hospice movement can be seen as an extension of that as people demand to be involved in decisions affecting their deaths, and those of their loved ones. The concept of the hospice and the ideas and practices that make up the hospice-care philosophy have existed for hundreds of years. In fact, the history of the word "hospice" implies that there may have been a time in our pre-industrial past when this "innovation" in caring for the dying patient was standard practice (Saunders, 1976). What is new, though, is the bringing together of these elements into an integrated, self-conscious approach to service provision, along with efforts to make this kind of care widely available.

The modern hospice began as an alternative to caring for dying patients in hospitals or nursing homes and, in many ways, conforms to the notion of a "contradiction." A major issue facing hospices, however, is whether they want to, or can, continue as contradictions, or whether they should assume another relationship with the major institutions in this field. One way to address this issue is to identify ways in which hospices contradict traditional care-giving organizations, and what is involved in retaining these characteristics as increased size, funding, and utilization create pressures to modify or abandon the organizational and service innovations already realized.

## THE HOSPICE AS ALTERNATIVE INSTITUTION

Advocates of alternative service approaches are particularly aware that the way in which a social service is provided can be as important as the substance of the service. Unlike architecture, in the social services function is more likely to follow form. The location and decor of a clinic, the use of appointments rather than mass queues, evening and weekend hours, meeting clients in private offices rather than open bays, provisions for individual and family participation in decisions about service goals and procedures can have as much impact on service outcomes as the competence of service providers. Kanter and Zurcher (1973) describe several organizational features which, taken together, form an alternative-service organization philosophy. Three elements of this philosophy relevant to hospices are: an emphasis on internal processes that promote wholistic approaches to service provision, power equalization and participatory decision-making, and small size.

*Process as product*. Like other alternative service organizations, an important value for hospices is commitment to certain organizational processes:

> The process of collective participation in decisions, the process of intimate communication with others, the process of crating a new kind of living space, the process of engaging in interesting work—these are the ends for which many alternative institutions strive. . . . [M]any alternatives value wholeness. They seek integration of life spheres; they seek to create work activities with family-like values . . . , to create situations in which the person can use all of himself—skills, resources, professional competencies, personal qualifications—and meet all of his needs—for creating, for working, for belonging, for meaning, for relating. (Kanter & Zurcher, 1973, pp. 390-393)

The current political environment, however, stresses service outputs rather than processes, particularly outputs that can be objectively measured. The shift from process to product is the result of the convergence of a number of constituencies within the social policy arena, particulary, fiscally-oriented policy analysts and program planners, and public managers with business backgrounds and/or training in business-oriented management schools.

This environment presents a serious challenge to hospice administrators intent upon maintaining an emphasis on program and organizational processes. The challenge centers on who sets criteria for judging program success or failure. It is here that the conflict between being a "poor copy" and a "contradiction" is sharpest. Are hospices to be evaluated along criteria established for traditional care facilities or are they to be evaluated along lines which reflect their unique characteristics?

Hospices, like most human service organizations, often have their goals defined by external bodies, particularly funding sources; these externally-set goals then become the sole criteria for assessing program effectiveness. This situation is exacerbated by the fact that highly-valued internal processes like broad-based participation in decision making, power equalization, and interdisciplinary teams, are often "loosely-linked," or completely unrelated to the goals external bodies are interested in accomplishing. Thus, a hospice charged with providing so many home visits or so many hours of counseling within a reporting period can accomplish this regardless of whether or not clients and staff are involved in decision making, or whether a team approach is used. In fact, research indicates that in terms of sheer productive efficiency—that is, the number of units of service per dollar expended, or the dollars expended per unit of service—the more bureaucratically organized the agency, the better:

> A heightened reliance on formalized rules and procedures apparently facilitates concentration of decision making power in the hands of a few. . . . Further, it is this concentration of power that facilitates productivity and efficiency. (Glisson & Martin, 1980, pp. 33-34)

However, the same research shows that bureaucratic centralization also contributes to staff dissatisfaction, a lower quality of client service, and a diminished level of worker and program development.

If hospice administrators are to protect and nurture valued internal processes, they must be presented as goals rather than means for accomplishing a goal; in short, the process must be a product. This is no easy feat under the best of circumstances, and it is especially difficult in the present political and social climate. Difficult as it is, however, it seems to be the only path. The alternative strategy—trying to show that these processes will contribute to greater agency productivity and efficiency—is often not realistic. In most instances, the goal of efficient production is not operationally connected to the practices that hospices are most interested in protecting.

Since one of the primary aims of hospices is to promote a set of alternative values around care for dying patients and their families, this must be presented as a philosophy of service with merit and importance in its own right. A strong case has to be made to the general public that in hospice work, as in international diplomacy, "the form is the content." Hospice administrators and staffs must continue to resist attempts to categorize valued internal processes as merely one of several possible alternatives for attaining externally-defined production goals; these processes must be presented as important values in themselves.

*Power sharing*. Many hospices seek to share power between administrators and service providers, among staff members (including volunteers), and between the organization and its clients. Concern with power sharing and broad-based participation in decision making assumes particular importance because of the emphasis on interdisciplinary teams and volunteers for providing services.

Any discussion of organizational power is hampered by the different meanings people give it. For many, power, whether in an organizational or societal context, means coercing others to follow the dictates of the powerful. Moreover, it is also assumed that people use power to promote their own interests at the expense of others. Another approach to power, however, sees it as the ability to get things done through directing resources and the activities of others toward goals that benefit all concerned. In this context, organizational power is, as Kanter (1979) suggests, analogous to physical power:

> It is the ability to mobilize resources . . . to get things done. The true sign of power . . . is accomplishment—not fear, terror, or tyranny. Where the power is "on," the system can be productive, where the power is "off," the system bogs down. (p. 66)

Increased concern over the distribution of power within organizations has prompted renewed interest in the nature of organizational power and the processes which create it. If we are to promote power sharing in organizations we need to understand why power is held by certain organizational members and not others, what can be done to alter the distribution of power, and what the consequences will be for organizational performance.

There is growing agreement that the major sources of organizational power are structural rather than individual. That is, an organization's design and production processes allocate considerable power to certain positions and little or none to others (Pfeffer, 1978). Factors associated with individual and unit power include location in the official hierarchy, performance of functions central to the organization's mission, and control over resources. This approach to organizational power injects a cautionary note into discussions of power equalization since it suggests that certain individuals and units *should* have greater amounts of power because of their location within the organization and the functions they are expected to perform.

A well-functioning organization should be able both to concentrate power in the hands of a few and disperse it among many depending on the situation. There are times when one person must be able to decide for the entire organization, as well as situations when a number of people, from various levels and functions, must have the ability to make decisions on their own. In order for power to be concentrated, organizational members must perceive that the person in whom power is concentrated is acting in the best interests of the organization as a whole. Conversely, for power to be dispersed, those at the top must view subordinates as capable of making decisions and able to be trusted with the responsibility of deciding on a course of action.

The distribution of decision making power in hospices is complicated by their limited autonomy due to dependence on externally-controlled resources. They are usually subject to extensive regulation by legislative, administrative, and community bodies. An example of this is the guidelines governing Medicare reimbursement (payment is authorized only when a patient is within six months of death) and their impact on how potential clients view hospice services. Lack of autonomy limits the degree to which organizations can develop services responsive to their clients' needs; instead, services often reflect constraints imposed by external forces, particularly funding bodies. Also, hospices frequently have imbalanced power relationships with hospitals (upon whom they depend for referrals) and the medical profession, which puts additional constraints on their ability to develop programs in keeping with their service philosophy.

Tensions can easily arise between top administrators and those in supervisory and direct service positions if the latter begin to suspect that administrators have been coopted by external forces and no longer represent the interests of the program. Conversely, when upper-level administrators suspect that others in the organization are doggedly pursuing narrow programmatic, professional, or personal concerns without an appreciation of the position of the organization as a whole, tensions and mutual distrust will arise.

One way of dealing with this situation is participation by all, or nearly all, organizational members in decision making. There are many advantages to broad-based decision making, particularly where it is essential that everyone's views be considered, or when everyone has information that bears on a decision. However, as with many things, too much of a good thing is not always desirable. Having everyone involved in all decisions can create more problems than it solves.

Participatory decision making is enormously time consuming, and when an organization must respond quickly and decisively, the necessity to consult large numbers of people puts it at a serious disadvantage. In addition, when making decisions most of us view the facts and alternatives from the perspective of the positions we occupy and the functions we perform. As the bureaucratic adage goes, "Where you stand depends upon where you sit." While there are advantages to having the people closest to a situation make decisions, there are also disadvantages, particularly when the issue to be decided upon has ramifications that go beyond the ken of the people closest to it.

An alternative for dealing with these concerns centers around the notion of organizational "cultures." One approach to organizational cultures is offered by Ouchi (Ouchi & Price, 1978) in his concept of "clan" organizations. Drawing on observations of Japanese industrial organizations, he defines a clan organization as a "culturally homogeneous organization, one in which members share a common set of values or objectives plus beliefs about how to coordinate effort in order to reach common objectives" (p. 36). Clan organizations have explicit policies on the goods or services to be provided, the technologies to be used, and appropriate organizational and administrative forms.

The clan organization socializes its members so that each merges individual goals with organizational ones. Through this process, organizational members acquire information on the "best" way to get things done, that is, the way most consonant with the overall organizational philosophy, thus making decision making almost instinctual. This socialization is possible, however, only when new members already share values quite similar to those of the organizational culture, which makes radical resocialization unnecessary.

In clan organizations the question shifts from who's making decisions to what decisions are being made—that is, regardless of where decision making power is located, are the outcomes of decisions in keeping with the organization's mission and values? Ideally, this enables every member of the organization to participate in all decisions through the exercise of oversight power. Administrators and staff alike are held accountable to a common set of criteria spelled out in the organizational mission statement.

The clan approach should be particularly attractive to hospice organizations since many already operate along these principles. Most people working in hospices were already committed to the hospice philosophy prior to becoming a hospice employee. The issue that faces the developing organization, however, is how to keep the organizational culture intact while responding to changing conditions and demands. To pursue the cultural analogy a bit further, just as there are historical societies that have not survived because of cultural rigidities that prevented them from adapting to changing circumstances, so are there organizations with similar problems (Hirschhorn, 1978). To prevent this, organizations must develop mechanisms for revising their philosophical and operational frameworks as the need arises (Torbert, 1985). An essential consideration in this is the importance of maintaining clarity about which are core organizational values that cannot be compromised and what can be modified or replaced without changing the character of the organization and its programs.

*Small size*. A final characteristic associated with most hospices is small size and the importance attributed to this. "To grow, stay small" is a slogan that could easily be adopted by many of these organizations. A size sufficiently limited to permit face-to-face relationships among all organizational members is valued because it is seen as the means for implementing other alternative values.

> Small size permits greater contact among all participants in a system. . . . Small size is seen as permitting more fulfilling human interaction, involving more widespread participation, and mitigating tendencies toward inequality. . . . [S]mall size can allow more attention to individual needs and loosen a reliance on standardized roles and responses. (Kanter & Zurcher, 1973, pp. 387-399)

While many equate bureaucratization with bigness, research has shown that small size by itself does not deter the growth of bureaucratic practices such as a strict division of labor based on functional specialization, a system of formal procedures dealing with work situations, and impersonality of interpersonal relations. Other factors that contribute to bureaucratization include the nature of the task to be performed, an organization's history, and the nature of the organization's environment (Hall, 1967). In particular, it has been suggested that organizations in environments with a "dominated external coalition," that is, organizations that are dependent upon one or a few external bodies for funding, accreditation, referrals, and the like, are forced to develop internal bureaucratic structures in order to cope with external demands (Mintzberg, 1984). As hospices become dependent upon one funding source (Medicare), the pressures to develop tighter management controls and formalized procedures mount. While limited size is not, by itself, a sufficient condition to retard the growth of undesirable bureaucratic practices, it is probably a necessary one. That is, while small organizations may be bureaucratically structured, large organizations must be. While hospices should take efforts to prevent growth beyond a point at which bureaucratic structures become inevitable, they must also be aware of other factors associated with the growth of bureaucratic procedures, particularly the administrative culture and the pressures and constraints arising from the environment.

## *STRATEGIES FOR ACTION: INTERNAL AND EXTERNAL PERSPECTIVES*

The foregoing discussion identifies several issues facing hospices as well as ways for addressing them. As with all service organizations, hospices must deal with internal matters concerning service provision and external factors concerning relationships with other organizations and forces in their environment.

A major internal concern is the ability of hospices to preserve their unique approach to serving the dying and their families, and the organizational and administrative forms developed to do this. Most hospices already have a clearly defined organizational culture subscribed to by most people who work in them, and many function like Ouchi's clan. However, the American hospice exists in a social and cultural setting in which the denial of sickness and death is an integral feature. Aggressive medical treatment and cure at any cost are the preferences of most Americans when faced with terminal illness. The notion of accepting and preparing for one's death is, at best, a "precarious" value in this society, to the extent that it is a value at all. The success of the hospice movement in the United States involves, as Kastenbaum (1977) suggests, a test "of the bonds of affiliation within our society. Do we have enough in common among ourselves to sustain the hospice? Or is the hospice a good idea that becomes—and remains—reality only under exceptionally fortunate circumstances?" (p. 231)

In order to preserve their service and organizational philosophy in what is often a hostile environment, hospice workers must become, in Selznick's (1957) words, "experts in the promotion and protection of values." Ways of doing this range from the gimmicky (McDonald's "Hamburger University," IBM's "company song"), to the personal and psychological (support groups and workshops on stress-management and burnout), to the philosophical, reflected in Ouchi's clan or Selznick's notion of "socially integrating myths" that "infuse day-to-day behavior with long-run meaning and purpose."

An important external task for hospices is to alter environmental forces unsupportive or detrimental to their service mission. These include community sentiments and attitudes, funding patterns, governmental regulations, and policies of other professional and service organizations. Most hospices have unfavorable power relationships with significant organizations in their environment, particularly funding bodies. The major strategy available to correct that, and one that hospices already engage in through federated state-wide associations, is the creation of coalitions. Through coalition-building hospices are in a better position, although by no means an equal one, to negotiate with powerful others for terms more favorable to their service goals.

Coalitions can assume varying degrees of commitment. At a minimal level, members share information by pooling the intelligence each possesses. The next step is to assimilate information, using pooled intelligence for diagnosing system-wide problems (What trends do we see? What problems are developing in the field as a whole?). The level of mutual consultation develops when member organizations consult with one another on problems that they individually face. This can lead to joint strategic planning where problems are identified that affect all member organizations and agreements developed on how they will be handled. Finally, a coalition can become a power bloc that develops bargaining positions and pursues tactics aimed at bringing about desired outcomes (Schlesinger & Oshry, 1984).

Each level of coalition development requires member organizations to make stronger commitments to each other and the collective effort, with consequences for each member organization's autonomy. Also, each step entails a greater involvement of member organizations in explicitly political activities such as developing a power base and pursuing aggressive strategies for achieving goals. Both of these activities, and particularly the latter one, have traditionally been shunned by human service professionals. The present political and social environment, however, is one in which the survival of human service programs in a form determined largely by the people who work in and are served by them, makes political action a necessity (Weiner, 1984).

Freedom, it is said, exists in the "interstices of institutions." As our society becomes increasingly dominated by a small number of extraordinarily large and powerful public and private institutions, the ability of innovative organizations to maintain independence and develop according to their own lights becomes more problematic. The ability of the hospice to survive as an alternative for the terminally ill is one test of this proposition. While the hospice movement is a small one, its failure would have considerable symbolic importance for other organizations struggling to go against the tide. Its success, on the other hand, would be a much-needed sign that the age of "managementocracy" is not yet upon us.

## REFERENCES

Glisson, C.A., & Martin, P.Y. Productivity and efficiency in human service organizations as related to structure, size, and age. *Academy of Management Journal*, 1980, *23*(1), 21-37.

Hall, R.H. Organizational size, complexity, and formalization. *American Socio-*

*logical Review*, 1967, *32*(6), 903-912.

Hirschhorn, L. The stalemated agency: A theoretical perspective and a practical proposal. *Administration in Social Work*, 1978, *2*(4), 425-438.

Kanter, R.M. Power failure in management circuits. *Harvard Business Review*, 1979, *57*(4), 65-75.

Kanter, R.M., & Zurcher, L.A., Jr. Evaluating alternatives and alternative valuing. *Journal of Applied Behavior Science*, 1973, *9*(2/3), 381-397.

Kastenbaum, R.J. *Death, society, and human experience*. St. Louis: The C.V. Mosby Co., 1977.

Meyer, J.W., Scott, W.R., & Deal, T.E. Institutional and technical sources of organizational structure: Explaining the structure of educational organizations. In H.D. Stein (Ed.), *Organization and the human services*. Philadelphia: Temple University Press, 1981.

Miller, H., & Phillip, C. The alternative service agency. In A. Rosenblatt & D. Waldfogel (Eds.), *Handbook of clinical social work*. San Francisco: Jossey-Bass Publishers, 1983.

Mintzberg, H. Power and organization life cycles. *Academy of Management Review*, 1984, *9*(2), 207-224.

Ouchi, W.G., & Price, R.L. Hierarchies, clans, and theory Z: A new perspective on organization development. *Organizational Dynamics*, 1978, *7*(2), 25-44.

Pfeffer, J. The micropolitics of organizations. In M.W. Meyers and associates (Eds.), *Environments and organizations*. San Francisco: Jossey-Bass Publishers, 1978.

Saunders, C. St. Christopher's hospice. In E.S. Shneidman (Ed.), *Death: Current perspectives*. Palo Alto, CA: Mayfield Publishing Co., 1976.

Schlesinger, L.A., & Oshry, B. Quality of work life and the manager: Muddle in the middle. *Organizational Dynamics*, 1984, *13*(1), 4-19.

Seeley, J.R., et al. *Community chest: A case study in philanthropy*. Toronto: University of Toronto Press, 1957.

Selznick, P. *Leadership in administration*. New York: Harper & Row Publishers, 1957.

Torbert, W.R. On-line reframing: An integrative approach to organizational management. *Organizational Dynamics*, 1985, *14*(1), 60-79.

Weiner, H. Survival through coalition: The case of addiction programs. In F.D. Perlmutter (Ed.), *Human services at risk: Administrative strategies for survival*. Lexington, MA: Lexington Books, D.C. Heath and Co., 1984.

# Women Reaching Women: A Project on Alcohol and Other Drug Abuse

Diane Kravetz, PhD
Linda E. Jones, PhD

Largely as a result of the women's movement, there has been considerable redefinition of the needs of women substance abusers. The changing social circumstances of women in society at large gave rise to new groups of clients and workers who were intent upon placing women's unique concerns and needs as central aspects of services, programs and treatments for women. The grassroots efforts of women in their own communities were joined by the growth of Women for Sobriety, a national program for women abusers (Kirkpatrick, 1981; Sandmaier, 1980a; Schwingl et al., 1980).

As discussed by Miller and Philipp (1983), the alternative service agency often arises in response to such changing conditions, providing novel approaches to service delivery and innovative theories and techniques of intervention. As the political and social concerns that provided the impetus for the alternatives attain a level of mainstream acceptance, some of the goals and methods of alternative agencies are incorporated into established, traditional agencies.

This paper presents a case study of Women Reaching Women (WRW), an innovative program of services in Wisconsin concerned with the problems and needs of chemically dependent women. The program's goals, structure, and processes are grounded in feminist approaches and stem from feminist critiques of traditional services and treatments for women. Although the program is embedded in a

---

Dr. Kravetz is Professor and Director, School of Social Work, University of Wisconsin-Madison, 425 Henry Mall, Madison, WI 53706. Dr. Jones is Assistant Professor, School of Social Work, University of Minnesota, 224 Church Street, S.E., Minneapolis, MN 55455.

 

traditional agency, it operates relatively independently from the traditional network of services and maintains its "alternative" status. As a statewide, grassroots organization, WRW provides a creative model of service delivery whose success suggests its applicability for the delivery of services to other client populations.

The following analysis is based on findings from a study conducted by the authors of six alternative social service agencies in Madison, Wisconsin, which provide services to women and which incorporate feminist principles into their work. Agency documents, written questionnaires, and in-depth interviews were used to obtain information concerning the growth and development of these agencies over time and to assess the major issues and concerns that these agencies have confronted. For Women Reaching Women, information was obtained from the written questionnaire, from agency documents, and from 15 in-depth interviews with past and current Board members, staff, volunteers, funders, and service providers in other agencies.

## BACKGROUND AND MISSION OF THE AGENCY

The Women Reaching Women Project (WRW) is sponsored by the Wisconsin Association on Alcohol and Other Drug Abuse (WAAODA), which is a 20-year-old statewide, nonprofit, membership association. Members of WAAODA include people from business and industry, organizations and professionals in the fields of alcohol and other drug abuse and allied health and human services, and other concerned citizens. The agency provides public education and advocacy for the victims of alcoholism and other drug abuse and on behalf of those who work in the field. It also provides technical assistance to the alcohol and drug abuse field, local communities, schools, law enforcement agencies, the beverage alcohol industry, and to various health and human services.

The WRW Project began in 1978 as one of 28 Volunteer Resource Development Projects of the National Institute of Alcohol Abuse and Alcoholism and was continued under federal funding for four years. The federal money that supported WRW became part of the Block Grant process and, in 1982, the State of Wisconsin Office of Alcohol and Other Drug Abuse assumed funding responsibility.

The purpose of WRW is to make appropriate intervention and treatment services for chemically dependent women more available and accessible in the state through a statewide volunteer project designed to: (1) increase the effectiveness of efforts aimed at raising the public's awareness of the problem of women and alcohol and/or other drug abuse; (2) increase the effectiveness of efforts aimed at informing women of available services in alcohol and other drug abuse treatment and intervention; and (3) assist women in gaining access to service delivery systems.

WRW's mission, then, is to increase the numbers of women in treatment, to advocate for the needs of women in treatment, to promote healthy lifestyles for women, and to train and utilize volunteers to achieve these goals.

## *IDEOLOGICAL PERSPECTIVE*

> While women abusers comprise approximately 50% of the abusing population, only 14-19% are seen for treatment. . . . The project is focused on women because we believe there are many reasons a woman is dissuaded from seeking treatment for alcohol and/or drug problems. Among them are fear of losing her family, not enough money for treatment, and most important, the devastating stigma and blame which our society places on the woman abuser. (WRW materials)

Several core and interrelated women's issues define the philosophy of and need for WRW. Female abuse of alcohol and/or other drugs is understood to be related to women's social inequality, traditional female socialization toward dependency and submissiveness, and gender role conflicts. The underrepresentation of women in alcohol and drug treatment is attributed to: (1) the greater social stigma associated with substance abuse for women than for men; (2) the lack of appropriate treatment programs for women; and (3) the unavailability of child care.

WRW, as well as the literature on women and substance abuse, focuses on the fact that researchers, physicians, mental health practitioners, and other service providers have ignored the patterns and experiences that characterize women's use and abuse of alcohol and other drugs. Established philosophies and approaches have failed to recognize or take into account the different consequences of chemical dependency for women and for men. In addition, male-dominated and male-centered organizations, treatments, and services are viewed as significant barriers to women's seeking and obtaining appropriate treatment and services (Burtle, 1979; Corrigan, 1980; Eddy & Ford, 1980; Glynn et al., 1983; Sandmaier, 1980b).

These women's issues permeate the philosophy and services of WRW. They are clearly articulated in the initial justifications for establishing the project, in funding applications, in training workshops and conferences, in informational materials and brochures, and in interviews with staff and volunteers. A Chapter Coordinator detailed the issue clearly:

> They [traditional programs] use a male model for recovery . . . so issues of family violence, bulemia, anorexia, incest, rape . . . are not addressed in treatment. . . . And they [women] get discounted. . . . People say, come on, you're just trying to get off the track, your real issue is alcoholism or drugs and you don't want to talk about that, so now you want to talk about binging and purging. They won't address it.

A client-volunteer highlighted the differences between goals for women and men in treatment:

> I don't think helpless is the way we're supposed to remain. . . . A.A. started really as a male-based group and men needed to let go and not be so in charge, I guess. We're not brought up to be independent and so telling us we're powerless just eats right into that, and we need to learn how to become in charge of our lives.

The need for a feminist approach is articulated by another leader in the organization: "Without feminist principles, you can attempt to get more women into treatment, which is one of the goals, but you're putting them into a treatment system which is not set up to help them become healthy."

Although the leadership of WRW and many of the volunteers view themselves as feminists, WRW is not a feminist agency in several respects. WRW is sponsored by and housed within a traditional organization in a field that has long been male-oriented and male-dominated in its philosophies as well as in its organizations and services. Its membership consists of women who are drawn by the importance of women's issues to their lives but who vary greatly in their political perspectives and social values. As one Chapter Coordinator explained:

> In my county, it tends to be a little more conservative, so I shy away from even using the word feminist, because so many of my volunteers, their hair would just stand on end. I think that they don't realize that they support all those feminist issues.

Another Coordinator stated:

> When the word feminist is brought up to certain people, they really balk at that, so I really hesitate to use that word. . . . In terms of coordinators from all over the state, yes I do [use the word "feminist"]; but when I go back home, I'm real careful about what I say.

The central purpose of WRW is to provide needed public education, advocacy, and services in the field of alcohol and other drug abuse. In addition to the well-established complex of values and knowledge concerning substance abuse which are central to this field, for WRW, feminist theory and research influence their goals, structure, and services.

## *GOVERNANCE AND FUNDING*

WRW is coordinated by a statewide project director, who provides leadership, technical assistance and training to the 25 local county chapters and integrates all chapter efforts on a statewide level.[1] The WRW Project Director is the only full-time paid staff associated with this Project.

Several other staff of WAAODA are partially paid from WRW funds and serve some functions for the Project. The Executive Director of WAAODA gets a portion of her salary from the WRW grant. She represents the project to the WAAODA Board, the larger alcohol and other drug abuse (AODA) system in the state, and the legislative and planning bodies that are connected with project funding; and she holds hiring/firing authority over the Project Director. The Executive Director of WAAODA supervises the Project Director of WRW, working with her to set program direction, assess and pursue funding sources, and review ongoing project activities. The WAAODA Office Administrative Assistant and Secretary also receive some funding from the WRW grant and provide support services to the Project.

All major policies and goals of WRW must be approved by the

State of Wisconsin Office of Alcohol and Other Drug Abuse (the grantor), the WAAODA Executive Director, and the WAAODA Board of Directors. The Board consists of individuals whose commitment is to the field of alcohol and drug abuse, not specifically or necessarily to WRW. Not surprisingly, the Board represents a wide range of views concerning women, women's issues, and the importance of addressing the specific needs of women within this field; they mirror the range of attitudes toward women and women's issues that exist in the alcohol and other drug abuse (AODA) community at large.

The advantage of this structure is that in the process of tailoring and shaping goals and policies to address the concerns and political perspectives of the Board, WRW confronts early on the political and social realities of the AODA community in the state. In the process of defining and justifying their work in terms acceptable to a diverse Board, they also discover approaches that are more likely to be successful in the community. Also, being housed within a mainstream volunteer AODA association gives substantial legitimation and respectability to WRW, provides formal access and linkages to important agencies and networks, and enhances their stature with funding sources. As described by one early member: "Well, I was part of the larger organization, so I always sort of shielded myself with WAAODA. I didn't want to separate myself off; that was a problem that we were having already."

The disadvantages of this structure are evident as well. This alternative program must devote substantial time and energy in coping with survival within a traditional organization. In addition, they must share their funding from outside sources with staff who are only partially engaged with WRW efforts and who may or may not be supportive of the Project.

Every WRW chapter has an Advisory Board which is organized by the Project Director of WRW. Most Advisory Board members are professionals from the Alcohol and Other Drug Abuse (AODA) field and other human service agencies. Some are community leaders from other sectors of the community. The Board also includes at least one nonprofessional woman who has been part of the local AODA treatment system. The Advisory Board lends direction and support and helps the chapter be responsive to the political climate, resources, and needs of the local community. In addition to providing critical leadership, the Board gives credibility, visibility, and continuity to local chapter efforts.

The Director works with the Advisory Board to identify one or two individuals who would be interested in and capable of carrying out the responsibilities of the Chapter Coordinator. In some instances, an individual or group is interested in starting a chapter; here, one or two of these individuals may become the Chapter Coordinator(s) and be assisted in establishing an Advisory Board.

The Chapter Coordinators are responsible for integrating their WRW project within the county AODA system and for networking with local women's organizations. The Coordinators set yearly chapter directions, choose specific projects for the chapter, recruit and maintain volunteer staff, and seek funding for their chapter. Each chapter has a steering committee of volunteers which assists the Coordinator by assuming primary responsibility for specific chapter activities.

Currently, approximately, 300 women serve as volunteer staff of WRW. Most of these volunteers are nonprofessionals; others are social workers, physicians, pharmacists, etc. As in other alternative service agencies, clients and former clients assume important functions; in WRW, most of the women who serve as Coordinators and volunteers have been in AODA treatment, are significant others of abusers, or are adult children of abusers.

Although the Coordinators and volunteers are accountable to and work closely with the Project Director, they have substantial autonomy and flexibility. As explained by one Chapter Coordinator:

> One of the nice things about WRW is that we can do just about what we want to do in our chapters as far as how we set it up, how we run it, what particular projects we focus on. We have a pretty free hand.

When asked about decision-making in WRW, one volunteer stated:

> If you do not like something, you can complain about it, and do it openly. And if you want to take the initiative on yourself to change something, you can do that, as long as you stay within certain guidelines. . . . Everyone knows where the power lies but I don't think people are reluctant to speak out and say what they would like to see changed.

A Chapter Coordinator explained:

> When we received some funding for our project, the volunteers decided exactly how they wanted that spent. . . . I let the

women decide how they think it's best needed because these are recovering women themselves and they can best tell us where the money is needed right now and how it can best be spent within the community.

Formal and hierarchical lines of authority and power exist between the WRW Project Director, the WAAODA Executive Director, and the WAAODA Board. However, within WRW, power is decentralized, with much decision-making being done by the Project Director together with the Chapter Coordinators and Advisory Boards. Volunteers have significant input into program planning and priority setting in their local chapters and at training events, and through regional meetings and statewide conferences. Throughout WRW, there are strong feelings of shared responsibility and mutual support.

Chapters are often housed within local AODA service providers such as mental health centers and local AODA councils. Some operate out of women's centers; others out of women's homes. Those chapters with local sponsoring agencies have office space and some supplies. Many chapters, however, rely on their own local fund-raising activities, donations, and the ability of their members to provide gasoline, refreshments, stamps, envelopes, etc. Currently, four WRW chapters have Coordinators who are paid part-time through local county and/or agency funding. Most Coordinators serve on an unpaid basis.

## *FUNCTIONS AND SERVICES*

### *The Project Director*

The Project Director of WRW is responsible for establishing and providing training and technical assistance to WRW chapters throughout the state. The persons who have held this position (three since 1978) have been responsible for establishing the 25 county chapters of WRW, including selecting the communities for the location of new WRW chapters; training chapter coordinators; organizing new chapters through on-site visits and volunteer recruitment and training; and providing some funds for ongoing chapter support.

The Project Director holds regional meetings and conducts training workshops for Chapter Coordinators and volunteers to provide information and stimulate the sharing of ideas and concerns. Her training efforts include discussion of advocacy techniques appropriate for influencing treatment centers, local political organizations, and legislative issues; technical assistance on fund raising; and provision of information concerning current legislation and treatment issues. The Director provides technical assistance and training to local chapters concerning organizing and facilitating women's support groups for recovering women and linking chapters with community child care programs to help provide child care for women in treatment.

The Director also helps chapter public-awareness efforts by assisting them in preparing articles for local papers; in participating in local television or radio interview shows; in developing public service announcements; and in planning personal presentations to community businesses and organizations. She also works with chapters in organizing statewide women's conferences each year.

Training efforts are also directed toward raising the awareness of state AODA treatment program directors and staff concerning the special needs of women in treatment. This training program is organized in conjunction with the State Office of Alcohol and Other Drug Abuse and includes evaluation of current treatment programs and recommendations for change.

The Director coordinates her activities with other state organizations concerned with alcohol and/or other drug abuse among women. She works closely with two statewide women's groups, the Women's Alliance on Alcohol and Other Drug Abuse and the Wisconsin Women's Network. The Wisconsin Women's Network is a statewide political advocacy group around women's issues and is particulary focused on legislative efforts; the Wisconsin Women's Alliance is a coalition of women working in the field of AODA who are concerned with identifying and advocating for the alcohol and other drug needs of women.

One important factor for the success of the WRW Project appears to be the presence and effectiveness of the Wisconsin Women's Alliance and the Wisconsin Women's Network. These two political groups provide strong advocacy concerning women and substance abuse in the state. Their advocacy for women directly benefits WRW since WRW is the only women's project within the AODA treatment delivery system.

### Chapters

In general, chapters focus on "before treatment" and "after treatment" concerns, concentrating on bringing more women into treatment and providing the support necessary to assist a woman in being successful in her recovery.

The basic types of activities carried out by local chapters include speaking engagements; media campaigns; community outreach and networking; local and statewide advocacy; fund raising for their local chapter and for the statewide WRW Project; finding ways to provide child care for women in treatment; setting up First Friends projects in which volunteers offer support and accompany women who are newcomers to Alcoholics Anonymous, Alanon or Alateen; facilitating support groups for women who have completed treatment, are significant others of AODA abusers, or are adult children of AODA abusers; facilitating Women for Sobriety meetings and children of alcoholics groups; organizing programs for volunteers; and contributing to the statewide newsletter.

In addition to these basic goals for every chapter, local chapters are expected to be responsive to the particular needs and problems in their own communities. Wisconsin counties differ significantly in terms of their openness to and experience with women's issues. Chapter activities, goals, and strategies in the more liberal communities differ from those in the conservative counties of the state.

Some counties have significant numbers of ethnic minority and poor white women. In addition to the stigma attached to being a female abuser, racism and classism exacerbate women's isolation and create formidable barriers to their receiving treatment. Some WRW chapters have been organized to specifically address the needs of these women.

## DISCUSSION

Women Reaching Women's success is apparent through several measures, including its continued funding; increasing support from its sponsoring agency and board; growing membership; increasing acceptance from Alcoholics Anonymous, Alanon, and state agencies; growing interest in the WRW model from agencies across the country; requests for the Project Director to present at regional and national conferences; and the devotion, enthusiasm, and commitment of its leadership and members. Through grassroots organizing, WRW has built an impressive network that is readily mobilized to influence legislators and to provide services.

Through numerous individual contacts and meetings at the local level, WRW has been able to convince many Alcoholics Anonymous groups and AODA agencies of the need for such a project; and in many communities, they have begun to overcome the prejudices and stereotypes that services by women for women routinely encounter. They have alleviated fears of competition by stressing the ways in which WRW services increase access to and facilitate the work of other AODA groups. They have focused on those women's issues that have become part of the public domain and have taken into account the political climates of communities. As described by one early leader: "We helped initiate programs in the community that didn't look like we were terribly radical . . . like public education film showing. . . . Only later did we start putting together women's groups."

This alternative program merges forces and factors which are often viewed as antithetical to one another. It combines the strengths of professionals with those of nonprofessional volunteers and demonstrates that these two groups can work together. It merges feminist theory and practice with conventional services and knowledge bases. It maintains formal and meaningful linkages with both mainstream and women's organizations and has formulated a mandate that is broad enough to engage the support of the traditional power structure as well as the feminist community.

Throughout all of the interviews, respondents expressed dissatisfaction with the current funding level of WRW, especially with the lack of funding for local chapters. Volunteers were discouraged and angered by the stresses, both financial and psychological, that accompany insufficient funding. Volunteer turnover, that many defined as high, was often attributed to the fact that women's economic position requires their finding paid rather than volunteer work. Coping with volunteer turnover, dealing with the priorities and goals of sponsoring agencies across the state, and being enmeshed in a highly male-oriented and traditional field, constitute substantial challenges for this under-funded agency.

It appears, however, that the social and personal needs met by this project, the strong leadership of the Project Director, and the dedication of WRW members are sufficient to mediate the debilitating effects of these organizational difficulties. As expressed by the Project Director: "In spite of it all, in spite of all the struggles

. . . we're really making some strides, and I think we're really having an impact."

Respondents' concerns with high turnover, political tensions within sponsoring agencies and local communities, and insufficient funding were consistently paired with high motivation and commitment to the project. A woman who works in an AODA agency observed: "These women really cared about what happened to other women and that was really different than other human service agencies where the people do it because it is a job . . . [they are] very committed to the cause."

Another woman described the volunteers as: "Dedicated . . . nurturing, it's a real caring organization, real nurturing to one another. The support that they give to one another is very impressive."

Respondents consistently remarked on the high level of concern, encouragement, and support that exists among women in WRW. The continued and consistent growth of WRW over time and the content of the interviews both support the conclusion that intangible rewards, such as recognition and mutual support, have been sufficient to engage volunteers on an extended basis. Nevertheless, for the long-range survival of the project, there is consensus that the work of Chapter Coordinators should be compensated and that chapters need additional funding to support their activities.

Given the decline in government revenues and support for the human services, there is increasing attention to the methods and problems of cutback management (Bozeman & Shusher, 1979; Pawlak et al., 1983; Reisch & Taylor, 1983). It is increasingly apparent that social programs will have to develop new approaches to service delivery. As stated by Parham (1982), "We will be pushed to innovate – use volunteers, paraprofessionals, family and community networks, self-help groups" (p. 100). WRW offers a creative approach which integrates elements from several of these sources. WRW demonstrates the viability of extensive volunteer participation within the human services, with decentralization of authority and decision-making and considerable reliance on community networks and self-help groups.

Bombyk and Chernesky (1985) propose that "Beta style" leadership may be particularly useful for social service administrators during times of retrenchment. This alternative model of leadership is "reliant upon diffused horizontal power, and concerned with the sharing of resources, collective problem solving, and the establishment of interdependent and cooperative relationships . . . and special attention is given to the personal needs and feelings of staff members'' (p. 49). WRW serves as a concrete example of the viability and effectiveness of Beta style leadership. Since this model emphasizes maintaining a favorable workplace, the Beta style may partially account for the successful growth of WRW despite their under-funding and often antagonistic or disinterested environment.

Respondents in this study were optimistic about the future of this program. Some representative comments include:

> I think it will grow in terms of the number of chapters in the state. . . . I see their role as growing and expanding . . . as women become more self-assured and as men become more accepting, I think that the doors will open.

> People are looking for ways to maximize service with limited dollars, and that's what WRW does. It targets a female population with very few dollars and is very effective. So, yes, I could see it moving beyond Wisconsin.

> I do believe that it is a moving force and that it is going to get stronger.

Respondents knowledgeable of federal and state level funding uniformly asserted that, as public concern grows in support of services for chemically dependent women, WRW's service delivery model will attract national attention and receive a much deserved recognition. WRW's model, which provides public education, advocacy, training, and services through a statewide network of volunteers, offers many intriguing possibilities for other human services as they respond to the challenges of declining revenues and emerging social concerns.

## REFERENCES

Bombyk, M. J., & Chernesky, R. H. Conventional cutback leadership and the quality of the workplace: Is beta better? *Administration in Social Work*, 1985, *9*, 47-56.

Bozeman, B., & Shusher, E. A. Scarcity and environmental stress in public organizations: A conjectural essay. *Administration & Society*, 1979, *11*, 335-355.

Burtle, V. (Ed.). *Women who drink: Alcoholic experience and psychotherapy*. Springfield, IL: Charles C. Thomas, 1979.

Corrigan, E. M. *Alcoholic women in treatment*. New York: Oxford University Press, 1980.

Eddy, C. C., & Ford, J. L. *Alcoholism in women*. Dubuque, IA: Kendall/Hunt Publishing Company, 1980.

Glynn, T. J., Pearson, H. W., & Sayers, M. (Eds.). *Women and drugs*. Rockville, MD: U.S. Department of Health and Human Services, 1983.

Kirkpatrick, J. Women for sobriety. In D. Masi (Ed.), *Organizing for women*. Lexington, MA: Lexington Books, 1981.

Miller, H., & Philipp, C. The alternative service agency. In A. Rosenblatt & D. Waldfogel (Eds.), *Handbook of clinical social work*. San Francisco, CA: Jossey-Bass, 1983.

Parham, T. M. J. Social service issues and challenges in the 1980's. *Administration in Social Work*, 1982, *6*, 91-105.

Pawlak, E. J., Jeter, S. C., & Fink, R. L. The politics of cutback management. *Administration in Social Work*, 1983, *7*, 1-10.

Reisch, M., & Taylor, C. Ethical guidelines for cutback management. *Administration in Social Work*, 1983, *7*, 59-72.

Sandmaier, M. Women helping women: Opening the door to treatment. In C. C. Eddy & J. L. Ford (Eds.), *Alcoholism in women*. Dubuque, IA: Kendall/Hunt, 1980a.

Sandmaier, M. *The invisible alcoholics: Women and alcohol abuse in America*. New York: McGraw-Hill, 1980b.

Schwingl, P. J., Martin-Shelton, D., & Sperazi, L. The first two years: A profile of Women Entering Women, Inc. In N. Gottlieb (Ed.), *Alternative social services for women*. New York: Columbia University Press, 1980.

## NOTE

1. For additional information concerning Women Reaching Women, contact Sharon Huggins, Statewide Project Director, WAAODA/WRW, 2801 West Beltline Highway, Madison, WI, 53713.

# PART 2: PUBLIC SECTOR STRATEGIES

## Administrative Entrepreneurship in the Public Sector

Paul R. Keys, PhD

Politics, administrative advocacy, entrepreneurship, and innovation are often not the guiding ideology of public sector human services agencies. Following a public administration model, many administrators place a high value on neutrality – non-involvement in partisan political affairs. At the same time, many public agencies dismiss innovation and advocacy efforts as too controversial, and detrimental to career longevity. The conventional wisdom is "don't rock the boat," "play it safe and avoid controversy." Since controversial agencies and agency executives sometimes do lose public support, these assumptions tend to go unquestioned. This paper is the account of a unique public human services agency, the Boone County Community Services Council, that defied these tenets, achieved a startling array of services innovations, and permanently changed the way in which human services were delivered for an entire community.

Dr. Keys is Associate Professor, Hunter College School of Social Work, The City University of New York, 129 East 79th Street, New York, NY 10021. The author wishes to thank Jim Bodard, former Executive Director of the Boone County Community Services Council, for his assistance in the preparation of this article.

 

## CRITICAL CONCEPTS

Recently, theorists familiar with operational needs of human service organizations have focused on administrative involvement in politics (Richan, 1981; Stern, 1985), the politics of social administration (Gummer, 1985) and the role of politics in public human services administration (Bevilacqua, 1985). An understanding of the applications of the "politics of administration" by social work administrators is essential. But for various reasons, both professional and philosophical, social workers frequently are unwilling or unable to apply political techniques to legitimate social work agency ends. Partisan politics and interest group politics are particularly difficult for both public administrators and social workers. Social workers who are administrators of public agencies thus encounter a double set of alleged value restrictions in using political power.

Equally relevent to this case study is the concept of administrative advocacy. As defined by Richan (1980), administrative advocacy refers to a leadership role of the social administrator, central to the administrative function, which sees a "vital connection between the organization's long-term self-interest and the welfare of . . . its clientele" (p. 73).

Palumbo, Musheno, and Maynard-Moody (1986) define entrepreneurship as a contemporary concept just beginning to be applied to public sector management. It is an important determinant of innovation in the private sector (Peters & Waterman, 1982). Private sector entrepreneurs who pioneered computer, technological, and telecommunications advances are characterized as risk takers – individuals who are alert to new opportunities, have the knowledge to exploit these new opportunities and are able to combine a number of production modes in new ways. Since 1985, entrepreneurship is also becoming accepted in public sector management (Lewis, 1984).

Innovation, while not a new term, is used in new ways in this analysis to suggest recommendations for new or revised programs that are qualitatively different from the status quo in an organization. The term is not necessarily equated with invention, in that the critical features of the recommended program may already exist in other organizations (Delbecq, 1978). A key feature of innovation seems to be the repackaging of existing concepts to create new realities – in this case service programs. The introduction of change is a key feature.

And finally, an understanding of demonstration projects is necessary for this case study. According to Vosburgh and Perlmutter (1985) demonstration projects provide practical experience with new programs or routines. However, it is essential to recognize that they are also political systems with a highly visible agency power base, with liabilities as well as advantages.

All of these concepts provide a theoretical basis for the discussion of the Boone County Community Services Council (BCCSC).

## *THE CASE STUDY*

### *Background*

Columbia, Missouri, with a population of 62,000, is the major city in central Missouri. It is the home of the University of Missouri system and is located in a rural, conservative, Republican part of the state called the "Little Dixie" area. The County of Boone, with a population of 40,000, is composed of five small incorporated cities. The County is primarily a rural farming community with pockets of industry. Except for the city Housing Authority, and the city's Youth Services Division, Health Department activities were the only human services activities conducted by the city and county before creation of the BCCSC. A number of voluntary social agencies, including affiliates of the major national agencies, service the city and the surrounding area.

The view that overlap and duplication by service providers existed were major local issues that led to the creation of the Boone County Community Services Council. Local political and community influentials of the two jurisdictions entered into an uneasy coalition and created the Boone County Community Services Council as a vehicle to accomplish somewhat contradictory local goals: (a) holding social services expenditures to a minimum through comprehensive public-private social planning, which would lead to elimination of the supposed gaps and duplications that "squandered" funds; and (b) at the same time favoring services deemed necessary by local elites.

Given the local situation, the BCCSC's mandate was a strong one: It was an organization created by local political consensus to address local social problems. It was, therefore, designated as the community's response to comprehensive social planning and coordination. There were no federal or state mandates and restrictions on program direction. It was a unique mandate as the organization received strong public and private sanction to "control" services.

Its formal mission, as defined in its charter, was to utilize citizen input to: (a) conduct a countywide social needs assessment study; (b) to develop a comprehensive human services plan to guide public and private human services funding; and (c) to coordinate efficiently the efforts and services of public and private agencies. Several related objectives flowed from the mandate: formal, on-site evaluations of local agencies receiving or applying for local funds; merging evaluations into city and county budget hearings and appropriations processes; "representing" agencies receiving favorable recommendations for city/county funds in budget hearings; and creating a directory of local services.

An eleven member Advisory Board, jointly appointed by the city and county, served as the governing board. While appointed by the city and county, the board set policy based on its own conception of community needs. Since the BCCSC was neither a city nor a county agency, neither its operations nor policy decisions were directly governed by the city, county, or United Way—a critical factor which created an opportunity for innovation.

The BCCSC was not only a research, planning, and evaluation agency but was recognized by radicals, liberals, the minority community, and student leaders alike as a promoter of social action and community change. It was probably this, more informal aspect of its program, that caused the BCCSC so many local political problems. There were constant political public attacks on the BCCSC, usually from county leaders, timed to surface during hearings on the BCCSC's budget. However, the BCCSC, with press and community support, usually decisively won these battles and emerged even stronger. The following describes the strategies used by the BCCSC as it made innovations and engaged in entrepreneurship activities that continue up to the present. It is the social work practice stance that is addressed in this paper.

## Strategies

### (1) Political

BCCSC strategies for change centered mainly around the use of traditional political techniques in a nontraditional setting, that of a public human services agency. The agency promoted social change by building political alliances with various radical, liberal, and minority groups in the City of Columbia. In addition, through conscious planning in the charter, influential board members (e.g., the Governor's Press Aide) and the local media were in effect brought into the coalition.

An early agreement of the BCCSC board, in writing the charter, was that all records would "always be available to the press at all times." The BCCSC approached press relations as a strength, sending materials to the press on a weekly basis and regularly meeting with reporters, editors, and editorial boards. The press, having details of the BCCSC's program and systematic cultivation, responded by giving consistently favorable news coverage. Another factor was that the BCCSC was controversial, and on slow news days good for a "filler" story. In crises, the media could also be counted on to offer support. In a sense, the BCCSC developed the status of a reliable news source by giving numerous "off the record" tips to the local media which then gave the BCCSC what it needed—air time, news stories, and favorable editorials.

For example, the Executive Director learned that the chair of the County legislative body planned to criticize strongly the BCCSC as a "waste of taxpayer dollars" at its session the next day. After a hurried session with the President of the board, a comprehensive listing of BCCSC accomplishments to date was drafted. At the legislative session, the list was presented to the county and press in the form of a press release. One of the items listed publicized a request to the BCCSC by the county chair for assistance with a study of county reorganization, specifically for an analysis of the options for a paid, professional, county administrator. Headlines that day and the next focused not only on the *pros* and *cons* of such a paid county administrator but questioned why the county was "keeping the study a secret." The original question of BCCSC's worth was permanently forgotten in the subsequent week-long press battle between the County Chairman and the media.

Traditional social work community organization skills were a part of the reason for BCCSC administrative successes in local politics. The Director typically "hit the streets" prior to each annual budget submission and secured a volume of letters of support from labor leaders, ministers, business leaders, favorable political leaders, and other local influentials. This is, as suggested by Ecklein and Lauffer (1972), the planner as "concert master," maintaining and building program support—an indispensable activity for any administrator in the public eye. The United Concerned Citizens

(UCC) is the best example of these community organization approaches. In this instance, the minority community was developed as a major component of the agency's constituency and was the lead partner in a coalition of students, radicals, and liberal, local influentials of both political parties.

In 1975, the BCCSC Director organized an underground, minority action group, known as the Columbia United Concerned Citizens (UCC), stemming from weekly luncheon meetings with the sole black city council member.

The luncheon meeting rapidly expanded to include ministers, and other minority leaders from the Housing Authority, city Youth Division, Board of Education, and private sector, among others. Eventually, the meetings moved from a local restaurant to become a weekly brown bag lunch in a local black church. Here, a plan to lobby appointments of minorities to city and county advisory commissions was developed. Few minorities had ever been so appointed. Lists of qualified minorities were compiled, and the entire UCC and their friends and families strategically wrote letters of support as appointments were considered. The result was success in 29 of the 35 appointments supported. UCC persons were appointed to major commissions such as Community Development Block Grant (CDBG) that recommended major local funding.

The UCC technique was never to identify itself formally; rather its efforts surfaced as a "spontaneous" collection of individual citizens supporting a given issue or appointment. The first minority appointment as Assistant City Personnel Director was through the UCC lobby process. An unrealized UCC agenda, however, was to unite with student coalitions and support student and minority candidates for City and County government posts.

The minority agenda also provided legitimate objectives for the program, as affirmative action was by statute in all of the demonstration funds used by the BCCSC. A minority radio show was another example of meeting the needs of the constituency. In addition to entertainment, it served the political purpose of providing a public forum for viewpoints of the BCCSC's minority supporters.

Research, through a Needs Assessment, was used in an innovative way to provide a scientific basis for BCCSC recommendations. By thus legitimizing its recommendations, the BCCSC made them much less subject to attack in the political arena.

A Mayor's Consortium was another example of positive use of

politics by the agency. The BCCSC, through Community Development Block Grant funding, helped the county's five mayors secure tangible resources for their cities (e.g., a water line, fire hydrants, a sewer extension), all valuable assets for their re-election campaigns. The mayors reciprocated by lobbying for BCCSC programs and budgets with the BCCSC's most unstable funding source, the county, and were a force that could not be ignored by county political leaders in making countywide budget decisions.

*(2) Advocacy*

Advocacy is almost inseparable from the use of political activities to advance public agency agendas. In one sense, in public human services administration, the administrator, especially the social work administrator, must have strong values and a sense of purpose for the agency and its clients. Frequently, these values are at odds with those of political superiors or elected officials. It is the use of politics and advocacy that allows these agendas to be "safely" accomplished by the sophisticated administrator. Here, there was a strong commitment to direct resources to previously powerless groups through BCCSC human services plans and administrative funding recommendations. There are risks for the administrator to take this type of position, but the risks are offset to a large degree by the strength of coalitions, local influentials, and constituencies developed through the advocacy process. This was precisely the case with the BCCSC.

For example, the BCCSC was a major advocate for an "alternative," volunteer counseling group, the Everyday People (EDP), that sponsored emergency shelter and counseling for street people, drifters, alcoholics, and drug abusers. EDP was almost totally a student volunteer operation, but effective with a group not served by mainstream agencies. Everyday People also operated a 100-watt F.M. alternative radio station. Due to a clash with conservative, midwestern lifestyles, the EDP never received public funds for any of its activities. The BCCSC recommended the group for funding, supported its FCC application for license renewal, and attempted to help it secure state and foundation funding for appropriate parts of its program, while protecting its advocacy functions.

The BCCSC (pre-cable T.V.), through UCC, addressed the issue of lack of a communications vehicle in Columbia's minority community and attempted to start a minority newspaper; "mysteriously" the major daily newspaper then offered a weekly full page devoted to minority news. The BCCSC approached local television stations and secured voluntary agreements to televise minority programs such as "Soul Train." Everyday People's radio station allocated five to six hours each Saturday afternoon for a minority DJ program giving air-time to minority news, music, and other interests. These were important contributions to the quality of life for the city's minorities, and also helped communicate events and activities.

*(3) Entrepreneurship*

Development of Title XX funding to implement the comprehensive plan (developed as a result of the Needs Assessment) is perhaps the best example of BCCSC entrepreneurial activities. Leveraging its initial $29,000 budget and combining it with city funds given to support other local human services functions, the BCCSC through Title XX was able to develop almost one million dollars in new services in less than fifteen months. Twenty-four local agencies were funded as part of the comprehensive plan, following upon the BCCSC Needs Assessment.

Moreover, Community Development Block Grant funds, in addition to supporting the Mayor's projects, were approved for helping a UCC affiliated group develop a minority shopping center. Through BCCSC technical assistance, almost $100,000 was allocated to support planning and acquisition of a site. Lastly, Comprehensive Employment and Training Act (CETA) funds were secured for many local agencies through efforts of the BCCSC, the newly-hired Assistant City Personnel Director, and the UCC.

*(4) Innovation/Demonstration*

The construct of innovation might be viewed as diffused throughout the BCCSC's political, advocacy, and entrepreneurial activities; it was a keystone of the Title XX-funded demonstration project. Title XX and other block grant funds were creatively linked to local human services programs in new ways that enhanced local human services and client needs. It was, irrespective of conservative local attitudes, the prospect of new sources of local funding and the ability of the BCCSC to understand and direct these new revenues that enabled the organization to foster so much local change. It was the demonstration project that was the source of local political power for the BCCSC.

## *IMPLICATIONS FOR SOCIAL WORKERS*

Social workers often view administrators as passive, bureaucratic agents of the status quo; rarely is there a recognition of the usefulness, skills, and position of the administrator as a force for positive change (Neugeboren, 1985; Richan, 1980). The BCCSC example illustrates how formal, public organizations may be uniquely used, consistent with professional principles, to achieve controversial community goals. The BCCSC consciously cultivated and utilized local influencing techniques and approaches to achieve human services ends of improved and expanded client services.

Moreover, the approach illustrates the close relationship between community organization skills and effective administrative practice. Finally, the BCCSC case counters the notion that administrators must "play it safe" in order to succeed. The BCCSC was the recipient of numerous state and national awards for its local human services planning efforts; among these was a commendation from the Missouri General Assembly, and a Horizons on Display National Award from the U.S. Department of Housing and Urban Development for the 1976 Bicentennial, as an example of local planning for the year 2000 (Horizons on Display, 1976). A framed, handwritten plaque was also given to the organization by Everyday People.

The role of the demonstration project as a base for innovation, advocacy, and change is affirmed by the BCCSC experience. Much of the initial leverage available to the agency came about as a result of its ability to innovate and demonstrate complex, new systems of resource allocation. The BCCSC was alert to the implications of these systems and, in a sense, was an early pioneer of entrepreneurship in the public sector, acting as a broker between the vertical systems outside Columbia and the horizontal local systems in the community (Merton, 1966).

Advocacy, entrepreneurship, innovation, and change, contrary to general expectations, may be promoted by public agencies that create appropriate local conditions. A prerequisite is an understanding of the use of political power and a commitment to positive social change. This is the account of such a local agency in a conservative, midwestern community that achieved a remarkable amount of advocacy and social change in a short period of time.

## REFERENCES


Bevilacqua, J.J. State politics is the name of the game. In F.D. Perlmutter (Ed.), *Human services at risk*. Lexington, MA: Lexington Books, 1985.

Delbecq, A.L. The social political process of introducing innovation in the human services. In R. Sarri & Y. Hasenfeld (Eds.), *The management of human services*. New York: Columbia University Press, 1978.

Ecklein, J.L., & Lauffer, A.A. *Community organizers and social planners*. New York: John Wiley & Sons, and the Council on Social Work Education, 1972.

Gummer, B. The social administrator as politician. In F.D. Perlmutter (Ed.), *Human services at risk*. Lexington, MA: Lexington Books, 1985.

*Horizons on display: A catalogue of community achievement*. Washington, DC: American Revolution Bicentennial Administration, and the U.S. Department of Housing and Urban Development, 1976.

Lewis, E. *Public entrepreneurship: Toward a theory of bureaucratic political power*. Bloomington, IN: Indiana University Press, 1984.

Merton, R.K. Local and cosmopolitan influentials. In R.L. Warren (Ed.), *Perspectives on the American community*. Chicago: Rand McNally & Co., 1966.

Neugeboren, B. *Organization, policy, and practice in the human services*. New York: Longman, 1985.

Palumbo, D., et al. Public sector entrepreneurs: The shakers and doers of program innovation. In J.S. Wooley, et al. (Eds.), *Performance and credibility: Developing excellence in public and non-profit organizations*. Lexington, MA: Lexington Books, 1986.

Peters, T., & Waterman, R.H., Jr. *In search of excellence*. New York: Harper & Row, 1982.

Richan, W.C. The administrator as advocate. In F.D. Perlmutter & S. Slavin (Eds.), *Leadership in social administration: Perspectives for the 1980's*. Philadelphia: Temple University Press, 1980.

Richan, W.C. *Social services politics in the United States and Britain*. Philadelphia: Temple University Press, 1981.

Stern, M.J. The politics of American social welfare. In F.D. Perlmutter (Ed.), *Human services at risk*. Lexington, MA: Lexington Books, 1985.

Vosburgh, W.W., & Perlmutter, F.D. The demonstration project: Politics amid professionalism. In F.D. Perlmutter (Ed.), *Human services at risk*. Lexington, MA: Lexington Books, 1985.

# Creating an Alternative Work Culture in a Public Service Setting

Marie Weil, DSW

Of all possible settings for alternative programs, the large bureaucracies of the public human service sector are typically viewed as the least likely and most inhospitable. The large scale and complex hierarchies, coupled with funding and operational constraints of the public sector, contribute to the judgment of conventional wisdom that if innovative, alternative programs are to be developed, private or grassroots agencies present the best options. In many instances that judgment is true. However, where there is a convergence of necessary preconditions, including internal and external environmental support, organizational readiness in relation to technology (Hasenfeld, 1983) and leadership with the vision, creativity and power to plan and champion an innovation, it is quite possible to develop alternative demonstration programs in large public bureaucracies.

This paper presents a case study documenting an innovative, alternative program serving highly vulnerable clients which was established in one of the largest county departments of social service in the nation – the Los Angeles County Department of Children's Services Child Sexual Abuse Program (CSAP). The program development and stabilization process offers guidelines for establishing an alternative program with a collaborative, feminist-oriented organizational sub-culture within the structure and hierarchical culture of a massive bureaucracy. The program's focus on building a partnership with self-help client groups – chapters of Parents United – and its focus on treatment and empowerment of victimized children and their mothers demonstrate the efficacy of a collaborative service planning and delivery model in creating positive change in the

---

Dr. Weil is Associate Professor, School of Social Work, University of Southern California, University Park, Los Angeles, CA 90007.

 

lives of clients. The matrix management structure and staff interaction patterns illustrate one means to empower staff and humanize the work setting for social service professionals operating in an intensely demanding and stressful service area. Analysis of CSAP's development, of its leadership succession, and creation of a functional, flexible, collegial culture reveals a model for effective alternative program development in the public sector.

## *CONCEPTUAL ANALYSIS*

Three conceptual issues are useful in analyzing the particular conditions which enabled a positive outcome for the public sector alternative program: (1) an emerging feminist approach to child welfare services; (2) alternative and feminist leadership and management approaches; and (3) the creation of a collegial organizational culture and felicitous leadership succession. Relevant points from these areas will be used to highlight issues in alternative program development.

### *Emerging Feminist Approach and Child Welfare Services*

Sexual abuse of children has increasingly been recognized as an extremely serious problem in American society. Media coverage of sexual abuse issues has increased reporting of incidents; however, the rate and severity of sexual abuse is also escalating throughout the nation (Gillies, 1986). Programs to deal with sexual abuse and treatment of offenders and victims are burgeoning, but there are inherent problems with the theory and research initially used as a basis for program design.

It is only recently that feminist issues and feminist analysis have been applied to child welfare services. As Costin (1985) points out, "a feminist perspective applied to the child welfare system can clarify illogical rationales that underlie the unequal status of mothers in an authoritarian family structure and the purposes that have been served by centuries of confining women to an oppressed and dependent status" (p. 197).

Many families in which incest takes place are almost stereotypes of patriarchal/authoritarian control in which the father's rigidity and the family's isolation further the breakdown of nurturing and appropriate parental roles. Curiously, much of the literature on incest and sexual abuse has followed the destructive pattern of blaming the mother and sometimes the child victim for the incest and abuse enacted by the father (Wattenberg, 1985).

Because of their research designs, theoretical models and treatment approaches, the early medical/psychiatric research studies easily identified the wife as the "silent collaborator" if not arranger of incest (Wattenberg, 1985). This explanation of the etiology of incest and much of the research conducted in the last two decades seems designed to fulfill the myth rather than to examine the actions of the perpetrator. Incest becomes another way to claim (as did Adam) "The woman made me do it," thereby exonerating the incest-committing father. In examining the rise of this myth of maternal collusion in incest, Wattenberg (1985) conducts a feminist analysis and recasts "the drama of father/daughter incest within the reality of a patriarchal system" (Costin, 1985).

An analysis which identifies the need for empowerment of women to enable them to protect their children from incest requires a model of practice which focuses on empowerment of women and children who have been victimized. Such a focus demands reshaping treatment of incestuous fathers as well as their families. Empowerment models for clients and novel staff collaboration with self-help groups, however, are unlikely to work unless the staff also feel empowered as professionals.

### *Feminist/Alternative Management Approaches*

Creation of an alternative management approach within a public bureaucracy requires strong leadership within the program and equally strong administrative support within the agency hierarchy. It is possible for an alternative program to develop through benign administrative neglect, but the continuance of such a program is always at risk that it will attract attention and be subsumed into standard operating hierarchical procedures. A management system which can be described as alternative and feminist consists of the following components: (a) flexible teams with leadership based on expertise for particular task accomplishment; (b) mutual planning and problem-solving among all professional staff during regularly scheduled meetings; (c) strong emphasis on process and consensual decision-making among professional staff; (d) nonhierarchal staff relations; (e) an empowerment focus employed with clients, self-help groups and staff; and (f) all carried forward through a matrix management model.

This internal program structure reflects the management orientations discussed in the developing feminist social administration literature (Chernesky, 1980, 1986; Ellsworth et al., 1982; Hooyman & Cunningham, 1986; Weil, 1986a, 1986b). These developing models stress valuing women's perspectives and process, democratic structuring, and power-sharing. They also recognize that feminist-oriented programs typically have problem-solving, decision-making, and communication systems that employ consensual processes internally but use formal communication and hierarchical status as necessary in dealing with bureaucratic organizations (Hooyman & Cunningham, 1986; Weil, 1986b).

### *Leadership and Program Innovation*

Leadership, as well-documented in the organizational behavior literature, is a critical factor in program innovation (Hasenfeld, 1983; Hersey & Blanchard, 1984; Perlmutter & Slavin, 1980; Schein, 1985). Two issues are significant in analyzing its impact on the Los Angeles Child Sexual Abuse Program: leadership style and succession.

*Leadership style* is the sum of the characteristics which shape the ways someone exercises leadership and guides decision-making in an organization. It evolves from an individual's personal style and personality traits influenced by culture and socialization and is molded by education, theoretical models and trial and error experience. Schein (1985) identifies three competency areas as aspects of leadership style: analytic, interpersonal and emotional. For feminist-oriented administrators, leadership style will be honed to reflect concerns for process, power-sharing and consensual decision-making.

*Leadership succession* refers to the changes in leaders which may or may not meet developing program/organizational needs. Increasingly, organizations are being analyzed in terms of "life cycle" issues. Kimberly (1980) identifies the stages in an organization's life cycle as "initiation, innovation and institutionalization." Organizations may experience a succession of leaders at different life cycle points or an individual leader will need to adapt management emphasis in accordance with the demands of successive program development stages. Patti (1983) identifies specific developmental goals and management tasks related to program development stages—design, implementation and stabilization. This analysis of

CSAP examines leadership succession through a four stage model of program development: (1) design or initiation, primarily involving program planning, resource acquisition (Patti, 1983), establishing credibility within the parent organization, and demonstrating program potential; (2) establishment, which builds on plans and delineates the service domain; (3) implementation including development of staff organizational structure and competent program performance; and (4) stabilization, creating a functional work culture (Schein, 1985), and stabilizing internal and external relations and structure.

## THE CASE STUDY: THE LOS ANGELES CHILD SEXUAL ABUSE PROGRAM

In 1977, a task force of members of the Los Angeles Inter-Agency Council on Child Abuse and Neglect (ICAN) appointed by the Grand Jury and the County Board of Supervisors recommended establishment of a local public agency program to respond to the service needs of the growing number of children who had been sexually abused. The task force urged the development of a service model stressing psycho-social treatment, the development of a "strong self-help component," and professional case management for children who were victims of incest and their families (Gillies, 1982).

In 1978, the Child Sexual Abuse Program (CSAP) was established with one supervisor, one clerk, and six Master's level Children's Services Workers all of whom were experienced protective service workers with the county. The joint focus on treatment and involvement with self-help groups was drawn from the national pilot Santa Clara County Child Sexual Abuse Treatment Program (Giarretto, 1982). The Los Angeles program, however, was the first "attempt to implement a child sexual abuse treatment program within a large metropolitan community" (Gillies, 1982). Professional staff participated in two weeks of specialized training at the Santa Clara Project Center; and ongoing staff development, including weekly staff meetings, mental health consultation, and twice yearly retreats, remained an important element of the program (Gillies, 1982).

Several factors set this project off as atypical in California public social services. First, the strong external support from ICAN, which had considerable political clout and support from departmental administrators, created a positive environment and sanctioned the use of resources for innovative program development.

Second, the strong recommendation of the task force and departmental acceptance of the creation of a Master's level program staff (most of whom obtained clinical licenses while working in the program) was a major departure in staff deployment patterns. Key administrative support for this professional level of service has remained strong. At its inception, staff for the program volunteered – a factor which demonstrated commitment and willingness to be involved in planning and implementing an innovative service.

Third, the pattern of leadership changes illustrated both the necessity of strong and visionary leadership to establish an innovation and gave evidence of an appropriate succession of leadership styles to assure program implementation, growth and stabilization.

### *Empowerment of Staff and Clients*

Empowerment of both the woman/client and professional staff is at the core of a feminist/alternative management approach. CSAP was revolutionary for the county in its commitment to empowering staff through shared planning and decision-making and matrix management, and empowering clients through the development of self-help groups.

#### *Changing Staff Responsibilities and Participation*

The triune CSAP commitment to provision of basic child welfare services and case management, provision of psycho-social treatment to child victims and their families, and creation and staffing of self-help groups of Parents United was indeed a tall order. The beauty of the model was its recognition of the critical importance of each of these service components in building an alternative and empowering service system for clients who were often isolated, victimized and dysfunctional. As the program moved into full implementation, the service model with restricted caseloads was adapted to focus on group treatment as both a particularly effective service modality for the target population and a cost-effective delivery model.

Initially, staff provided an array of services including case management, crisis intervention, protective services, dependency court investigation services, dependency supervision services, and individual, conjoint, and family therapy to targeted families within a specified geographic catchment area stretching from Pasadena to Long Beach (Gillies, 1982).

As caseloads increased, it became impossible for CSAP staff to carry forward case management, child welfare and group treatment services along with intensive individual and family therapy. The solution was to affirm group treatment for parents, victims and siblings as the treatment of choice for CSAP clients. Other therapeutic services were referred to public or private agencies where clients paid a fee for services. Group treatment within CSAP remained free of charge.

With program evolution several modifications were made in staff responsibilities. The responsibility to carry out initial protective service investigations was removed from the demonstration program and relegated to regular child protective services staff. This reallocation removed the burden of intensive initial investigations. That relief was counterbalanced by the increased necessity to work collaboratively with protective service staff throughout the county.

In addition, staff worked with Parents United leaders to strengthen their organizations and enable them to offer crisis intervention counseling. As the program developed, it became necessary clearly to separate treatment from case management roles. To prevent role blurring and client confusion between treatment foci and the necessarily authoritarian role related to court appearances, a decision was made to assure that parents were not placed in therapy groups which were led by their Children's Services Worker.

With program stabilization, basic responsibilities for each professional staff member included: (a) coordinating at least one Parents United or Daughters and Sons United self-help program; (b) providing group therapy following self-help meetings; (c) providing intake and screening services; (d) coordinating case activities and planning case management for limited caseloads with family members, Children's Services Workers and Probation Officers; (e) providing community education, inservice training, and case consultation; (f) supervising and training professional volunteers; and (g) assisting in program development for the entire CSAP operation.

Staff empowerment in exercising these functions was carried forward through a collegial and feminist-oriented matrix management structure and process. Each worker was in charge of developing and coordinating activities with one self-help group. Functional leadership was shared depending on particular tasks and expertise. All staff were involved in weekly planning and decisions-making sessions, and treatment and action teams handled program tasks and internal, interagency and intergroup relations. Each worker was simultaneously autonomous in dealing with her own program area and part of a collegial planning and decision-making team. Both power and decision-making were shared. The high degree of direct service staff autonomy and planning responsibility are rare especially in public sector program development.

By September 1982, after the program had moved to focus on group therapy, 440 clients per week were receiving service in 32 therapy groups. In late 1983, over 600 clients were participating in 45 therapy groups. The number of parents participating in Parents United programs throughout the county has currently stabilized to between 600 and 800 persons (Gillies, 1986).

As clients increased and as workers became responsible for providing treatment through an ever increasing number of Parents United groups, program leadership responded creatively to a crisis of worker overextension. The program for professional volunteers was established to assure that all families in the program had access to treatment.

### *Involvement of Volunteers*

Professionals, many of whom were already licensed, and others who were seeking involvement and clinical supervision to qualify for state licensing volunteered to work as therapists in CSAP groups, adding a unique component to the Los Angeles program. Volunteer positions were also opened to graduate student interns and to volunteers from the Departments of Children's Services and Probation. All volunteers had to complete successfully the orientation and application process for acceptance into the program, were required to make a six-month commitment to the program and had to participate in ongoing training and supervision. Familiarity with the skills in employing the unique service model was assured through this intensive process. By the end of 1984, CSAP was supervising over 56 volunteer staff and 10 Special Projects staff—therapists who are employed by other agencies which have agreements to serve CSAP clients.

## *Self-Help Component: Empowering the Client*

Chapters of Parents United (PU) constituted the self-help component for adults through CSAP. Daughters/Sons United was the self-help component of the treatment program for adolescent sexual abuse victims and their siblings, and Children United specialized in group work with children between five and 12 who have been sexually abused. For younger children, play therapy and other modalities were employed.

The Los Angeles CSAP/Parents United partnership is complex. Local PU groups meet weekly for business meetings led by elected members who are officers of the self-help group and then CSAP staff lead group therapy sessions. "Parents United is a private, non-profit self supporting organization composed of the adult members of families where children have been sexually abused" (Gillies, 1984). The Los Angeles Chapters are affiliated with the National PU group. Local groups organize their own functions, determine what will occur at their weekly business meetings and carry out tasks. Each local group has officers and is responsible for its own fund-raising.

In 1981, a leadership training program was established by CSAP to provide training to parent members in crisis counseling so that they can function as a support network for each other within each of the chapters. A unique feature of the Los Angeles program is a representative PU County Council which meets regularly and sponsors seminars and an annual conference. Jointly, local chapters co-sponsor and operate the Los Angeles County Parents United Hotline, and members are prepared to provide community presentations. In all areas except therapy, parents control their organization, but all therapy group leaders are professionally trained – CSAP staff or professional volunteers. Within CSAP group treatment is highly structured and controlled and is based on support of external control systems – the Juvenile and Criminal Courts.

The partnership between officers of Parents United and CSAP staff has gone through an expected group development process. The chapters were initiated by CSAP staff and as local chapters develop, some conflict related to efforts to establish role definition have been inevitable. Clarity has been attained by establishing that parents are responsible for all Parents United organizational functions and business meetings, and that CSAP staff are responsible for leading the group therapy sessions. The troublesome question of "Who is in charge here?" with its attendant defensiveness was transformed by skillful leadership into the appropriate and enlightening query, "Who is in charge of *what*?" (Gillies, 1986).

The focus of the Parents Untied self-help groups and CSAP group therapy is designed so that perpetrators must acknowledge their own actions and their own responsibility. Self-help groups typically are quicker than professional therapists at cutting though excuses and rationalizations because they have "been there." One CSAP staff member reported that involvement with Parents United speeded up the therapeutic process related to acceptance of responsibility by an average of two months (Davis, 1985).

The groups are also an empowering force for mothers. Many women involved in Parents United have previously had little or no validation for functioning as autonomous adults. The group process fosters this development and helps them learn how to assert themselves and how to protect their children. Feminist-oriented program models, like CSAP, can assist in reshaping child welfare practices and interventions. Such practice models can be most effective when the operating organizational model and work culture support and live out, as CSAP does, the same values that are imbedded in the practice model.

## *Leadership Succession and Culture Creation*

The CSAP program presents an excellent case example of issues of leadership succession and creation of an alternative work culture in a large public setting.

### *Leadership Style and Succession*

While much of the organizational behavior literature specifies top level decision-makers only as leaders and counts others as managers/implementers (Schein, 1985; Bennis & Nanus, 1985) it is important to consider the role of supervisor/coordinator in this project as a bona fide leadership role. Despite the constraints of structure and procedure in large public agencies, program flexibility can be attained by those who have personal power within a system, who are viewed as competent and loyal, and who know the rules well enough to bend them to a point of strain but not fracture (Gillies, 1986). Such leaders are able to develop zones of creativity and community responsiveness within rigid hierarchies. Heads of special programs, if they are creative and organizationally savvy, may be able to exercise as much flexibility as if they were operating in the private sector – if they maintain program effectiveness and satisfy the political concerns of sanctioning bodies and high level administrators.

Each of the first three leaders involved in bringing the program from inception to stability had qualities of vision, creative problem-solving and organizational change know-how. All were MSW's who had front-line experience in protective services, dependency court proceedings and interagency liaison. The first program leader was eminently skilled in inter- and intra-organizational relations. She was politically astute, a creative and collaborative problem-solver and acutely aware of the importance of maintenance of external support from the Inter-Agency Council on Child Abuse and Neglect and the County Board of Supervisors. Her major leadership emphases were on basic program development and establishment of external political environmental support relations.

Her successor had considerable experience in mental health services and engaged primarily in development of connections with inter-agency direct service networks. She had skills in media relations and concentrated on development of the public image of the program. She emphasized the importance of maintaining CSAP as a separate entity – in the spotlight as a demonstration with national public social service implications. She was able to establish the program, market it and render it a force to be dealt with in inter-agency relations.

The third coordinator/supervisor faced the tasks of building the program, developing all areas of operations, and stabilizing it. She emphasized staff support and development, creation of needed policies, procedures, information management, collaboration strategies and internal administrative supports as well as continuing the inter-agency and political thrust to assure external environment support. Her leadership enabled the program to gain momentum, grow and stabilize and to become that rarity in public programs – a fully functioning, alternative work culture within a major bureaucracy.

### *Culture Creation*

The first coordinator had the personal, internal and external political power to garner support and induce the designed and recommended change in an established and rigid organizational structure – necessary factors for program initiation (Kimberly, 1980).

The second coordinator was able to establish the presence of the organization and gain acknowledgement of its existence in the service environment. The third maintained a flexible and innovative development style and at the same time was able to build, institute and stabilize policies and procedures. Most importantly, she nurtured and established the supportive, collegial work culture which undergirds this unusual program combining: (a) child welfare case management, (b) group treatment for families where incest has occurred, and (c) support for a strong client self-help/program partnership.

## *IMPLICATIONS*

The CSAP offers a transferable model for humanizing high stress service areas through its focus on empowering clients and its feminist-orientation to services for sexually-abused children, their siblings and parents. Within a large bureaucracy, programs can reframe their practice approach so that they function with shared decision-making responsibility, mutual participatory planning and problem-solving, and mutual dependence. Such restructuring requires a strong commitment to empowerment and mutual aid, for staff as well as clients. Beneficial results can accrue in reduction in the incidence of burnout for workers involved in this stressful service area, an increase in self-esteem and functional ability for mothers and child victims of abuse, and a lessening of the sense of isolation of dysfunctional families where trust between parent and child has been violated as a result of incest and sexual abuse.

The ability to maintain an alternative/feminist model internally and function in more expected formalistic ways externally is a much needed characteristic for feminist administrators (Hooyman & Cunningham, 1986). Leadership must be strong and flexible, capable of using the "hybridized" management style described by Lenz and Meyerhoff (1982), that is, using a feminist model internally through a consensual problem-solving approach, and regular administrative and bureaucratic skills in advocating for clients and staff with the external, complex larger system.

The creation of a high commitment work ethos, difficult to achieve in a massive public bureaucracy, is the responsibility of internal program leadership. This can be accomplished through ongoing in-service training and support, constructive and sympathetic supervision, peer group support, team decision-making and matrix management models.

Acceptance of a "life cycle" analysis of organizational evolution requires that leadership be responsive to the changing stages and needs of the program. Perhaps the most critical factor in developing positive stabilization for a program is developing capacity for assessment and change. As Kimberly (1980) notes, programs which cannot change and transform will eventually fail to be responsive to evolving environmental conditions.

The work culture in the Child Sexual Abuse Program illustrates the opportunities for development of feminist and alternative orientations even in large bureaucracies through leadership within specialized programs, units and work teams. The model offers an efficacious means to humanize a high stress workplace through collegial interaction patterns and matrix management.

## REFERENCES

Bennis, W.G. False grit: The myth that says you've got to be macho to get ahead. *Savvy*, 1980, 43-47.

Bennis, W.G., & Nanus, B. *Leaders: The strategies for taking charge*. New York: Harper & Row, 1985.

Bricker-Jennis, M., & Hooyman, N. (Eds.). *Not for women only: Social work practice for a feminist future*. Silver Spring, MD: National Association of Social Workers, 1985.

Chernesky, R.H. A new model of supervision. In N. Van Den Bergh & L. B. Cooper (Eds.), *Feminist visions for social work*. Silver Spring, MD: National Association of Social Workers, 1986.

Chernesky, R.H. Women administrators in social work. In E. Norman & A. Mancuso (Eds.), *Women's issues and social work practice*. Itasca, IL: F.E. Peacock, 1980.

Costin, L.B. (Ed.). *Child Welfare, Special Issue: Toward a Feminist Approach to Child Welfare*, May-June 1985, *64*(3).

Davis, A. Supervising children's services worker, L.A. county. Personal interview, May 1985.

Ellsworth, C., et al. Toward a feminist model of planning for and with women. In A. Weick & S.T. Vandiver (Eds.), *Women power and change*. Washington, DC: National Association of Social Workers, 1982.

Giarretto, H. *Integrated treatment of child sexual abuse: A treatment and training manual*. New York: Science and Behavior Books, 1982.

Gillies, E. Los Angeles county department of children's services child sexual abuse program. Biennial report. Los Angeles, 1986.

Gillies, E. Los Angeles county department of public social services child sexual abuse project—January 1978 to June 1982. Los Angeles, 1982.

Gillies, E. Executive Director, Southern California Training Center. Personal interview, July 1984.

Hasenfeld, Y. *Human service organizations*. Englewood Cliffs, NJ: Prentice-Hall, Inc., 1984.

Hersey, P., & Blanchard, K. *Management of organizational behavior: Utilizing human resources*. (4th ed.). Englewood Cliffs, NJ: Prentice-Hall, Inc., 1982.

Hooyman, N., & Cunningham, R. An alternative administrative style. In N. Van Den Bergh & L.B. Cooper (Eds.), *Feminist visions for social work*. Silver Spring, MD: National Association of Social Workers, 1986.

Kimberly, J.R. Initiation, innovation, and institutionalization in the creation process. In J.R. Kimberly & R.H. Miles (Eds.), *The organizational life cycle*. San Francisco: Jossey-Bass, 1980.

Lenz, E., & Myerhoff, B. *The feminization of America: How women's values are changing our public and private lives*. New York: St. Martin's Press, 1982.

Patti, R.J. *Social welfare administration: Managing social programs in a developmental context*. Englewood Cliffs, NJ: Prentice-Hall, Inc., 1983.

Perlmutter, F.D., & Slavin, S. *Leadership in social administration: Perspectives for the 1980s*. Philadelphia: Temple University Press, 1980.

Schein, E.H. *Organizational culture and leadership*. San Francisco: Jossey-Bass, 1985.

Wattenberg, E. In a different light: A feminist perspective on the role of mothers in father-daughter incest. In, *Child Welfare Special Issue: Toward a Feminist Approach to Child Welfare*, May-June 1985, *64*(3).

Weil, M. Women, community and organizing. In N. Van Den Bergh & L.B. Cooper (Eds.), *Feminist visions for social work*. Silver Spring, MD: National Association of Social Workers, 1986a.

Weil, M. Women in administration: Leadership and organizational culture. Invitational paper presented at the 1986 Community Organization and Social Administration Symposium, CSWE, Miami, March 9, 1986b.

# PART 3: INDIRECT SERVICES

## Administration of Diversity

Robert Fishman, MSW

Many social agencies can be described by the services they provide (e.g., the family service or adoption agency, the hospital or the mental health agency). By contrast, with more than seventy different projects ranging over numerous fields, Resources for Human Development, Inc. (RHD), in Ardmore, PA, cannot be adequately described by the projects it supports. Rather, as an administrative mechanism, it is unique in the combination of its diversity, structure and particular value system. RHD demonstrates the viability of an organization model that is designed specifically to encourage the entrepreneurial spirit, social responsibility, and creativity of individuals and groups in the community.

After sixteen years of development and with a current yearly revenue of over six million dollars, RHD is a model for other human service organizations. RHD is interested in demonstrating an effective humanistic new model for corporate structure. As a diversified nonprofit organization it administers a broad range of units including: out-patient mental health; methadone and alcohol services; residences for the retarded, mentally ill, homeless and alcoholic; transportation for the handicapped; workshops for the retarded; concerts in homes for the elderly, and a federal Head Start program.

A corporate "unit" is formed whenever a new source of funds,

Mr. Fishman is Executive Director, Resources for Human Development, Inc., 120 W. Lancaster Avenue, Ardmore, PA 19003.

 

for a new activity, is received. Therefore, a unit with its own director is established if five-hundred dollars is received from a foundation to begin an advocacy group of parents with deaf children, or if a governmental contract for three-hundred thousand dollars is received to establish a shelter for the homeless. In either case, the director of the unit is answerable to the executive director and his/her staff and makes all the programmatic and financial decisions indicated elsewhere in this paper.

In order for a corporation to support such innovative activity there must be high level support and value placed on innovation within the corporation. The writings of Peters and Waterman (1982) emphasize that most successful corporations in the private sector include support for innovation. They particularly note that:

> if you want to understand the culture that encourages entrepreneurial activities at 3M, as good a starting point as any is its value system, in particular, its "eleventh commandment." It is: "Thou shalt not kill a new product idea." The company may slow it down. Or, it may not commit a venture team. But it doesn't shoot its pioneers. (p. 227)

Such support for entrepreneurial creativity is rare in the nonprofit field, and yet the need for improvement and new ideas for the delivery of service is as great as in the private sector. The lack of financial reward itself does not stop such creativity – organizational reluctance does.

This paper will highlight the underlying value system and structure of RHD so that other corporations can embrace the model as a means of ensuring their own success at a time when the human service field is under such stress.

## *A CASE EXAMPLE*

The unique qualities of RHD are best illustrated by the "New Beginnings" project which is designed to attract people with new energy and new ideas into the organization. Anyone from the larger community can call if they have an interest in furthering a new idea which will provide benefit to others. The new potential not-for-profit entrepreneur is offered a meeting with a corporate executive within the same week. If the idea seems at all feasible, and the individual or group is willing to work on its development without pay, RHD offers office space, telephone and xerox use, and above all a range of consultation services. In addition, a modest sum of three-hundred dollars is offered to the new project to cover the cost of stationery and other minimal start-up costs. Recently, the New Beginnings project was reviewed in a local newspaper and over forty people called to share and brainstorm their interests; six new projects came to fruition as a result of that one article.

### *Setting the Direction*

RHD was born in 1970, when the newly formed corporate board and its executive director agreed to develop a new form of nonprofit agency: one that would experiment with structure. With an assurance of a grant of fifty-thousand dollars to establish an outpatient mental health service, the board and executive decided on the following:

1. That the board would hire or fire the executive, but delegate all other hiring and firing to that executive.
2. That the board would not provide a fund-raising function for the agency but that the executive and staff would be responsible for such funding and all day-to-day activities of the corporation.
3. That the board would review corporate policy decisions, the work of the executive and the maintenance of the financial integrity of the corporation, but would not form any standing committees and would not be involved in day-to-day decisions.
4. That the purpose of RHD would be to provide an open, creative and humanistic environment for a wide variety of services. That the inclusion of a new type of service would require acceptance by the board, but would be considered acceptable provided that the service contributed to the common good.

Aside from the above agreements RHD is, in many ways, similar to other human service organizations. It is incorporated as a 501c3 nonprofit; it has a standard set of bylaws; it obtains a yearly outside audit of its activities; and that audit is reviewed by the board.

### *Corporate Philosophy*

Any human service organization operates according to a set of values whether or not these values are made explicit. Ouchi (1981) emphasizes the importance of explicit corporate philosophy and argues:

> The bedrock of any Z company is its philosophy. . . . Philosophy and business are the most compatible of bedfellows. . . . A philosophy can help an organization to maintain its sense of uniqueness by stating explicitly what is and isn't important. It also offers efficiency in planning and coordination between people who share in this common culture. (p. 111)

For many years, RHD's value system has been a matter of conscious decision-making. As such the values are presented as a set of assumptions when the corporation is described to others and the values are included in RHD's corporate brochure. RHD feels strongly that the leadership and staff of corporations should endeavor to clarify value assumptions, and ask whether the structure of the organization and the behavior of its employees, particularly the corporate board and executive staff, are consistent with stated values. Only by being explicit about values involving specific behavior can an organization legitimately expose itself to criticism. Where it exists, corporate philosophy rarely identifies values about specific interpersonal behavior, yet it is at just this level that the human issues, the feelings we have about ourselves and each other, emerge in the workplace. As human service agencies, it would seem appropriate that we stand for affirming healthy behavior in our own work environments.

RHD's values statements are taken seriously, and indeed the following list is stated in our current brochure:

1. Human beings are of equal worth, regardless of race, creed, sex, or handicap;
2. We deserve to work in an environment that affirms our worth and avoids demeaning judgments;
3. We deserve the opportunity to express our creativity, while affirming the creativity of others; the corporate structure most conducive to these beliefs has maximum decentralization and local autonomy;

4. By responding to the basic good in people, the corporation maximizes individual commitment and responsibility; and,
5. A working environment which reflects these beliefs will be successful. (1980)

The statement of belief also affirms:

> The people of RHD share a common belief that by responding to the basic good and strength in people, we have our best chance of maximizing positive individual commitment and responsibility. We find this applicable when dealing with our employees, recipients of services, and other individuals with whom we are in contact through our many corporate activities. (1980)

Over the years, independent researchers have looked at the organization and interviewed unit directors as well as line staff. Consistently, employees have reported on commonly held corporate values. They recognize that the leadership of any one unit may behave in contradiction to the corporate value system, and consequently, at times, unit employees will challenge unit leaders or corporate office staff when behavior is seen as unacceptable. Recently one such challenge was brought to the executive director. A staff member reported the inappropriate behavior of a unit leader who "talked down to me and made fun of me in front of others."

When these and other complaints were heard by a long-term employee, she knew that such behavior on the part of leadership was inconsistent with corporate philosophy and observed, "That is not the way things are done at RHD and you can bring that complaint to the executive." This employer challenge led to further evaluation and the ultimate resignation of that particular unit manager.

In practice, this philosophy means that senior staff are there to encourage, assist, support, educate, and allow people to make commitments and assume responsibilities. It means trusting an employee to do his/her job and believing in his/her potential to take on even more difficult tasks. It means allowing a client to attempt growth which may seem risky, but knowing that the gains from the attempt (successful or not) will outweigh the stagnation of the status quo.

Given this belief system, when corporate staff challenge the authority of a unit director with regard to his/her programmatic decisions, that challenge takes on a particular meaning. RHD comes face to face with the fact that one cannot delegate and at the same time control behavior. Therefore, one must be clear about when behavior at the unit level can be challenged at the corporate level.

While RHD's statement of values does not change behavior itself, it provides a guideline for the evaluation of staff and leadership. Against that guideline, individuals can validly challenge each other. One can hear these values in action when people are overheard saying, "that's not the way we do things in RHD."

But, inevitably, differences do emerge between people and conflict is a part of corporate everyday life. RHD believes that corporate leadership must be explicit about the ways to deal with conflict.

### *Development of Internal Structure*

During RHD's first years of growth, decisions were made that affected internal structure, and that further differentiated RHD from other corporations. RHD was interested in encouraging face-to-face working groups which allowed employees to know who made the decisions that affected their daily work lives. Although it was clear that one could not avoid conflict, RHD was organized so that conflict could be dealt with directly by the people involved. Therefore, the executive and original staff agreed:

1. That each unit would be organized with an annual budget, a director and an ability to communicate directly with the funding source where appropriate.
2. That each unit director would hire and fire employees within that unit, and would set salaries within the budget and guidelines set up by their funding source and the executive staff of RHD.
3. That each unit director would provide policy direction for that unit as long as the activity satisfied the funding source, and the unit remained financially solvent.
4. That each unit director would have responsibility for purchasing.

By establishing these understandings, RHD eliminated the purchasing and personnel function in the corporate office and established those functions at the unit level. Most large organizations develop a middle-management level to handle and control such decisions. RHD rejected that structure because such decisions were to be made at the face-to-face level, and RHD wanted unit responsibility for the unit budget. To further the pattern of delegation to the unit level, it was clarified that salaries would be set on a unit by unit basis, depending on the funding stream and the unit's ability to stay within a balanced budget. Therefore, no corporate-wide salary scale exists today. Instead, each of the units and the corporate office, which is considered another unit, evaluates its financial condition and its needs and determines its expenditures.

Despite this decentralization, there is an automatic review at the corporate level, since all financial activities take place at the corporate office even though they are initiated by the unit director. There have been instances when we have found that a unit director has exceeded his/her delegated authority or initiated expenditures which were in conflict with a corporate policy or a government grant. At such times a meeting is immediately called and the problem confronted and resolved.

In delegating these responsibilities to an individual unit, the unit's identity is emphasized while the role that the corporate office plays in the day-to-day functioning of that unit is minimized; similarly, the corporate board minimizes the role it plays in the day-to-day functioning of the corporation. Understandably, units have developed strong identities and a sense that they are successful "businesses" committed to their clientele, their funding source, and their own integrity. To further this identity, it is expected that each unit will have its own name, its own brochure and stationery, and at times, its own advisory group. The energy and devotion that this creates in each unit is impressive. Unit leaders and staff demonstrate a commitment that would never develop if the unit were administered from a central corporate level. And the basic value underlying this structure is trust.

This supports the research of Peters and Waterman (1982), who found that successful corporations treated their workers with dignity and respect. Thus, the belief and trust in employees is clearly demonstrated when they are given the right to act without having to check most decisions at many different levels within the organization.

RHD has developed a horizontal organization without a middle-management level, and with day-to-day operational decisions delegated to the level. It has avoided the divisional directors who are in charge of purchasing, personnel, out-patient services, residential services, and research. The corporate structure of RHD may be diagramed as follows:

BOARD

CORPORATE OFFICE

UNIT UNIT UNIT UNIT UNIT UNIT UNIT UNIT

Thus, each unit is responsible for a broad array of functions which include both programmatic and support services. This also supports the findings of Peters and Waterman (1982) regarding the effectiveness of a simple corporate structure.

> A wonderful example of simplicity in form despite size is Johnson & Johnson. This company represents an extreme of keeping the structure simple, divisionalized and autonomous. As we've seen, J&J is a $5 billion company broken up into 150 independent divisions, average size just over $30 million. The divisions are each called "companies," and each of them is headed by a "chairman of the board". . . . Even though none of the companies is truly independent in the sense of having stock of its own, the "boards of directors" are active and buffer the divisions from unwanted (and usually unneeded) corporate interference. (p. 309)

RHD's commitment is to human needs, not pieces of machinery. The inability to make unique and variable decisions hampers the care of human beings who continue to display unique needs. Corporations will continue to serve their own structure rather than the people who come to them until they change those structures to fit the needs of those they are there to educate or help.

***Financial System***

In order for RHD leadership to track financially this wide-ranging organization with its emphasis on unit identity and decentralized decision-making, a unique cost-centered accounting system was developed.

During its formative years RHD struggled to find a balance between delegation and central responsibility, particularly in the financial area. It was recognized that the lifeblood of a nonprofit corporation was its ability to account for the appropriate expenditure of public funds. Therefore, there was, and is, no debate about the need for auditable records. However, auditability was, and still is, the argument most often given by corporate staff or visitors to justify questioning the delegation of power or to suggest withdrawal of such power. Such debate usually confuses the need to track money with the tendency to doubt the judgments of others on the expenditure of those dollars. The following system has been designed to handle the tracking issue:

1. All contracts must be signed by the Executive Director or the Board President. (This function is sometimes delegated to another corporate executive.)
2. All funds received by units within the corporation must be deposited in corporate accounts.
3. Funds can only be drawn from accounts by corporate checks issued by the corporate office.
4. All expenditures are either allocated to unit accounts or to the corporate office accounts.
5. All unit directors get detailed computer reports on all expenditures and income relevant to their unit, monthly.
6. Unit budgets include an overhead percentage on expenditures. This percentage is the income to the corporate office and is based on negotiation with funding sources.
7. Charges from one unit are never allocated to another unit; and, therefore, everyone knows that when funding stops, a unit goes out of business.
8. When units create a surplus of funds, all these funds remain within the unit for use at the beginning of the next fiscal year. Such unit funds are not to be spent by executive or board decision. Unit directors may require executive approval for expenditures if the amount is substantial.
9. All units are expected to operate within budgets or on a balanced basis, with exceptions requiring executive approval. Units operating with a deficit can be closed by executive decision.
10. An annual audit of all corporation activity is performed by an independent accounting firm and reported to the corporate board. (1975)

Within these guidelines, seventy active units are in operation, with a combined budget exceeding six-million dollars. RHD has been successful in finding unit directors who work very hard with their staffs to keep their units' budgets balanced, since it is only when units are solvent that unit directors and their staffs control daily programmatic decisions.

Earlier, the issue was raised concerning corporate level questioning of decisions made at the unit level. This is reviewed as a central issue in this organization model, and the matter is dealt with as a part of the corporate philosophy.

### *Conflict Management*

The rules which govern our approach to conflict affect all other aspects of administrative style. At RHD, we openly recognize that while conflict is not desirable, it is inevitable. In an atmosphere that aims to attract forceful and creative individuals, differences can get stormy. And, in such storms, leadership must be clear about its role and must limit its actions so that they flow from corporate principles. RHD's corporate understanding is that when employees report to us about any conflict in which they are involved we can:

1. Listen with empathetic interest to what they are feeling.
2. Offer advice about how they can better manage that conflict.
3. Offer to meet with both parties in the role of mediator or facilitator.
4. Continue to recognize and respect that both parties perceive their own reality as correct.

But we cannot:

1. Take sides or act as though it is our role to decide that one person is correct.
2. Offer to champion one person's perception and confront the other ourselves.
3. Assume that there is a simple right/wrong solution to issues.

These are the rules of behavior which begin to define a technology for managing conflict. This technology can help managers deal with everyday varieties of conflict. It is important to note, however, that there are three types of situations that would trigger exceptions to the use of the above listed principles:

1. When the communication includes any indication of client abuse or neglect.
2. When there is any indication that corporate funds are being handled unethically.

3. When a corporate employee is endangering a relationship with a funding source.

In any of these three situations the individuals involved are immediately called into the corporate office, the situation evaluated, and, if necessary, administrative action is taken. It must be emphasized that such administrative action has been necessary only six times during the last seventeen years; thus, it has been a rare occurrence.

It seems fair and consistent that the same rules of conflict management apply to corporate officers and staff as well as to all of our employees. Therefore, when the corporate leadership is in conflict with a unit director all of the above rules of behavior apply. We are no longer running a corporation that depends on the preference or whim of board or corporate leadership. We are operating an organization that strives to follow certain principles of behavior—an ethics of conflict management. Schon (1983), who recognized the importance of management's handling of conflicting views, quotes a manager as saying,

> I feel good when I see that engineering and development, advertising and manufacturing, are really surfacing and talking about their differences. It's my job to keep the dialectic alive. . . . Once you have identified the conflicts, you see to it that they resolve them and that they let you know the results. . . . A manager's task is to make sure that such conflicts are neither suppressed nor circumvented. (p. 254)

At RHD, people complain about each other with some frequency, but most often the complainer does not want to confront the other directly. The complainer actually wants to convince an authority that the other is wrong, hoping that the authority will intervene. But that is impossible at RHD. When employees do wish to work out conflict directly, corporate staff facilitates face-to-face meetings and provides non-biased arbitration.

Certainly, such conflict management is more difficult when the conflict occurs between corporate staff and unit directors. It takes a conscious effort to behave professionally, and not according to whim, as management takes on the responsibility of power and leadership. To help leadership and staff remember the rules of conflict management, conflict involving a corporate staff person is usually mediated by at least three or more members of the corporate staff, and includes the input of other unit directors. Final authority still rests with the corporate executive, although that can be challenged to the Board. We believe that that authority which is exercised least is best.

## *IN CONCLUSION*

Resources for Human Development, Inc. is seventeen years old, but by many corporate standards, the corporation is still an infant. RHD has viewed its central purpose as the demonstration of an effective new humanistic model for corporate structure. RHD has much to learn regarding this alternative structure. And we recognize that other work groups are also trying ways to rediscover basic issues such as the enhancement of quality, human worth and commitment. We are quite sure that no particular corporate style is right for any two different groups of people, but we are convinced that certain organizational behavior is destructive to its group members. We are quite sure that individuals in corporations, like those in families, will come up with different views of how to approach problems; but we are also convinced that organizational structures which negate people and operate on the assumption that employees cannot be trusted, will not fulfill their potential for enhancing the common good.

## REFERENCES

Ouchi, W.G. *Theory Z*. New York: Avon Books, 1981.

Peters, T.J., & Waterman, R.H., Jr. *In search of excellence*. New York: Warner Books, 1982.

Resources for Human Development, Inc. *Corporate brochure*. Ardmore, PA, 1980.

Resources for Human Development, Inc. *Statement of principles*. Ardmore, PA, 1975.

Schon, D.A. *The reflective practitioner*. New York: Basic Books, 1983.

# Alternative Federated Funds: Resourcing for Change

Felice Davidson Perlmutter, PhD

Federated fundraising is a 20th century phenomenon which has played a critical role in providing support for private agencies in the voluntary sector. This mechanism has served several functions: In addition to its basic support objective, it has allowed for the fulfillment of noblesse oblige (Lubove, 1965) while it simultaneously has created a stairway to corporate heaven as young captains of industry used organized philanthropy to climb to the top (Seely, 1957). It also democratized philanthropy as it spread the base from a select few to many donors on all economic levels.

The efficiency and effectiveness of this mechanism were accepted with little question until the late sixties, when new groups emerged which questioned the social service establishment and the status quo. Although agencies working for social change were often excluded from community funds (Steiner, 1925), it was not until the 1970s that redress was sought as new strategies were attempted (Weisner, 1983).

> United Way faces challenges from a number of groups, including racial minorities and a network of women's associations, that contend it has a near monopoly over employee deductions for charity. They also complain that United Way apportions the money it collects to favor older philanthropies. (Teltsch, 1985)

The emergence of Donor Option programs and the development of Alternative Funds in the past decade merit careful attention. Donor Option programs provide a choice to United Way givers to designate specific non-member United Way agencies to which their

---

Dr. Perlmutter is Professor, School of Social Administration, Temple University, Philadelphia, PA 19122.

 

money should be allocated. By contrast, Alternative Funds have been organized as fundraising systems by nonprofit agencies working for social and economic justice who have not had access to, and/or who were deliberately excluded from traditional funding sources, including United Way (Davis, 1975; Wenocur, Cook, & Steketee, 1984).

Given the emergence of Alternative Funds (Bothwell, 1978; Cook, 1983), more information regarding this new force is needed. This paper presents a case study of Alternative Funds in Philadelphia.[1]

## THE PHILADELPHIA CONTEXT

Philadelphia is unique in its success in serving as the site of three active and successful Alternative Funds. Philadelphia is also the site of the largest United Way Donor Option program in the nation. And finally, Philadelphia is enriched by the presence of a Center for Responsible Funding which serves a vital advocacy and coordinating function for the Alternative Funds.

This activity may be due, in part, to the unique social history of the city. First, the dominance of social agencies in the voluntary sector is characteristic of the Northeast, and can be traced to the activity of the Charity Organization Society in the late nineteenth and early twentieth century (Wilensky & Lebeaux, 1958). Thus, social services have been traditionally delivered in private agencies and Philadelphians are accustomed to supporting these agencies through the philanthropic dollar, primarily raised by United Way.

Second, Philadelphia has been identified as a city with a liberal tradition, influenced by the small but active Quaker community (Baltzell, 1958). It also has an active community of socially concerned citizens who represent various ethnic backgrounds and who are often involved in political and social causes. Many of these progressive groups were disaffected as they were excluded from the major funding mechanism.

And finally, the successful growth of a Donor Option program may be related to a critical incident which occurred in 1980. *The Philadelphia Inquirer* reported an agreement between United Way and the Catholic Archdiocese of Philadelphia whereby agencies which in any way offered birth control, abortion counseling, or services opposed by the Church were to be excluded from United Way funding. Since Women's Way had applied for membership, it was turned down. This galvanized action not only from affected and potentially affected agencies, but also from the broader citizenry. It appeared that a fundamental violation had occurred in an organization which held communal trust and which yielded communal power. In response to the furor created by this report, the United Way implemented a Donor Option program.

These several factors may have paved the way for changing the culture of federated fundraising in the local community.

## *CRITICAL ISSUES*

The following dimensions to be examined in analyzing the agencies in this case study of Alternative Federated Funds are selected as critical in any analysis of a social welfare program (Perlmutter, 1969).

1. What is the *mission* of the organization? What are the underlying values upon which the mission is based?
2. What is the *target population*? What agencies are eligible to receive services (i.e., allocations)?
3. What is the *governance* mechanism? Who are the critical actors/the organizational elites? (Selznick, 1957)
4. What is the *resource strategy*? How is the fund supported and how does it assure autonomy and continuity? (Perlmutter, 1971)
5. How do the agencies deal with *controversy*?
6. How do these organizations *relate* to one another?

The case study will be organized by these critical issues as the experience of the agencies will be compared and contrasted. It is our assumption that we are dealing with an alternative system and that the focus of discussion is across agencies.

## *THE CASE STUDY: ALTERNATIVE FUNDS IN PHILADELPHIA*

### ***A. Identifying the Critical Actors***

The critical actors in this case study are the agencies which compose the alternative funding system. Three of the agencies serve a direct funding function. They are, in order of dates of incorporation, (1) *Women's Way* (July, 1976), (2) *Bread and Roses Community Fund* (August, 1977), and (3) *Black United Fund of Pennsylvania* (March, 1982). A fourth organization which serves the indirect but vital functions of advocacy, coordination, mediation and research, is the *Center for Responsible Funding*, incorporated in 1979.

Each of these organizations shares social and political concerns; yet each of these organizations is unique in its operations. Together they provide Philadelphia with a potent force for meeting unmet needs and for bringing about social change.

### *B. Understanding the Critical Issues*

The following discussion will be organized by the six issues identified earlier: mission, target population, governance, resource strategy, dealing with controversy, and interorganizational relations.

#### *(1) Mission*

A common theme permeates the mission statements of the four agencies under study: the focus is on social injustice, fundamental social change, and self-empowerment:

The goals of *WOMEN'S WAY* and its member agencies are "to empower women and to change attitudes, laws and institutions which perpetuate the problems faced by women and girls."

*BREAD AND ROSES* was founded "with the belief that social injustices are often a reflection of fundamental societal problems. In response, the fund supports organizations which are working to establish basic human rights where these rights have traditionally been denied."

*BLACK UNITED FUND* is a mechanism "to organize the human and financial resources of the black community to participate in improving the quality of life of our people. . . . Such efforts emphasize mobilization of leadership around common goals that stress self-help and minimizes social, political and economic differences within the community." In fact, diverse issues such as economic development, arts and culture, education, social services, housing, civil rights, and criminal justice are encouraged rather than minimized.

*THE CENTER FOR RESPONSIBLE FUNDING's* constituency is "those non-profit organizations working for social and economic justice in oppressed communities. . . . The purpose of the Center is to change in some fundamental ways the fundraising climate for our constituent groups." The Center for Responsible Funding is distinctly different from the direct funding agencies in that its role is one of advocacy and coordination for all nonprofit organizations vis-à-vis fundraising, including the three Alternative Funds.

The values which underline these mission statements reflect a belief in self-help and empowerment, a belief in the rights of those with alternative life-styles and sexual preference, a concern with discrimination and oppression, and a focus on a more equitable distribution of wealth and resources in our society.

While each program has a particular mandate and a particular constituency, these commonalities inform the total alternative funding system.

*(2) Target Populations*

A discussion of the target populations which are served by these funds will serve to establish the unique identity of each program.

*WOMEN'S WAY* not only supports women's services but requires that each member agency "must identify itself as a feminist/woman-controlled and managed organization which is working toward the betterment of women and must have a self-help philosophy." Pro-choice is a requisite ideological stance. There are nine member agencies which meet these criteria whose varied services include reproductive counseling, learning opportunities for low income women, services for victims of domestic abuse, gynecological and obstetrical services, career advisory services, legal counseling and law reform litigation, services related to unfair or illegal job practices, and services to victims of sexual rape or abuse. In addition, Women's Way has a discretionary fund which allocates grants to non-member agencies "which provide special services and/or advocacy programs to women." Some examples of funded special programs are housing aid for single mothers, general services to Hispanic women, residential support services to women who are substance abusers, and direct services and advocacy for older women.

*BREAD AND ROSES*, guided by the motto "Change, not Charity," targets its funding to "local advocacy organizations, with priority given to community-based organizations which have limited access to traditional funding sources because they are considered too small, too new or too controversial." The areas of activity of the recipient organizations include human and civil rights, peace and disarmament, women's rights, international issues, worker's rights, and environmental concerns. Direct services and economic development projects are supported only if linked to social change programs or community empowerment.

*BLACK UNITED FUND*, with a broad target population "supports projects which have a positive and continuous impact on the lives of black people in health and human services, education, criminal justice, arts and culture, economic development, leadership development and emergency needs."

*THE CENTER FOR RESPONSIBLE FUNDING* views its target population in a broader sense. On the one hand, it serves the various local funding agencies as it seeks to provide advocacy and to improve interagency cooperation among them; simultaneously, it views its target population as large employers who have payroll deduction programs. Thus, CRF works with the City of Philadelphia and with the Board of Education to gain and protect solicitation privileges for the Alternative Funds.

The target populations of the alternative fund organizations reflect their respective mission and mandate.

### (3) Governance

An issue of central concern, articulated by the agencies being discussed, is to protect the mission of each program. Consequently, the governance mechanism has required careful design and, when necessary, flexible redesign.

*WOMEN'S WAY* is clear in its intent to give member agencies an active role in policy making, compatible with its philosophy of empowerment. While the governing board consists of representatives from both member agencies and the community-at-large, care has been taken to ensure that the agencies have the majority of seats. Consequently, there are two representatives from each member agency of Women's Way and "a nearly equal number of at-large representatives." Since the criteria for member agencies are clearly delineated vis-à-vis the ideology and mission of Women's Way, this assures that policy will be set within the given framework.

*BREAD AND ROSES* is a membership organization composed of donors, volunteers and grantee organization representatives. It is unusual in that all members meet annually to elect two boards:

(1) the Board of Directors is responsible for all policy and procedural decisions except for those dealing with funding; (2) the Community Funding Board deals with all aspects of funding including applications, allocations, grant-making policy and procedural decisions.

Guidelines have been developed for both boards to ensure representation of people of color, women and sexual minorities; donors and grantees must also be represented. One staff member also serves on each board. To assure communication and cooperation between the boards, there are two seats from the Funding Board on the Board of Directors. Furthermore, the majority of members on the Funding Board must be community activists.

To assure a broad donor pool, any person who contributes $50 or more can serve on the Board. This is a critical stipulation since more than 50 percent of the donors are wealthy. Since Bread and Roses has a large cadre of very wealthy donors, it has thus dealt with the pattern of policy and control being unduly influenced by a small cadre of donors. However, it does recognize the special needs of its wealthy donors who are struggling with their ideological commitments, and it has an ongoing monthly group meeting to work with this special constituency.

*BLACK UNITED FUND* has a Board which sets Fund policy. Members are recruited from a broad array of local organizations and must be at least 18 years of age. "Members of BUF Board of Directors are recruited from the clergy, legal, social work, accounting, and business professions. In addition, BUF has an Advisory Board made up of community members that work on special projects, i.e., fundraising, and liaison with labor, churches, and community." The Board is also actively involved in program development for the Fund.

*THE CENTER FOR RESPONSIBLE FUNDING* is managed by a Board of Directors a majority of which are "representative of social change, community self-help or constituency controlled organizations. . . . a majority are representative of the women, Latino, and Black communities and of other oppressed communities. . . ." Among these members are ones with legal, financial, and fundraising expertise. More than 80 percent have been affiliated with an agency or group directly involved as consumer or beneficiary of the services of The Center for Responsible Funding.

"The board has full programmatic and fiscal control of the Center's activities" (CRF Report, 1982).

All the boards have mechanisms built-in for rotation of members. While the terms and mechanisms vary according to the particular needs of the programs, all are concerned with the representation of points of view which reflect commitment to the agency's mission.

In addition to the board members, the professional leadership must be examined as a part of the organizational elites. All four agencies have women as executive directors, who give extensively of their time and energy. The salary level of all these executives is not commensurate with their competence or function. It is clear that they are directly contributing to the survival of each of these programs.

*(4) Resource Strategy*

Careful thought has been given to the issue of resource development and resource allocation. As each of the funds has grown in terms of the resources at their disposal, an ongoing debate has ensued, especially since the growth has been dramatic (Table 1).

This discussion of resources will deal with (a) source of funds, (b) allocations, and (c) reserve funds.

(a) In regard to *source of funds*, while all three funds have attempted to diversify their base, it is important to call attention to the unique major strategies of each. Women's Way has put its major efforts into individual and corporate contributions including workplace campaigns; it has also become very sophisticated in fundraising events, with an annual dinner which attracts more than 1,400 attendees (and which cleared $105,000 in 1986). The major source of funds for Bread and Roses is from individual donors; in 1985 this

TABLE I. BUDGET SIZE OF PHILADELPHIA ALTERNATIVE FUNDS

| | 1977 | 1980 | 1985 | 1986 (Goal) |
|---|---|---|---|---|
| Women's Way | $80,434 | $130,260 | $769,930 | $869,525 |
| Bread and Roses | | $87,553 | $343,400 | $520,000 |
| Black United Fund | | $11,936* | $62,460 | $100,000 |

*(1982 Budget data, founding year.)

accounted for 70 percent of its funds. While Bread and Roses has more than 1,000 donors, it must be noted the fact that more than half of its donor income comes from a small number of wealthy donors is a critical reality (with gifts ranging from $500 to $10,000).

Black United Fund is most successful with payroll deduction campaigns from Federal, State, and local government employees; this is comparable to the experience of the National Black United Fund (Teltsch, 1984).

Each fund has made choices to maximize the strategy which works best, given its unique organizational context and capacity. Each fund is thus clear in setting its priorities vis-à-vis fundraising approaches.

(b) The *allocations process* again reflects differences in the three funds. Women's Way is unique in that it supports nine member agencies and also has a discretionary fund for annual grants. Contract relationships have been most clearly delineated between Women's Way and its nine member agencies. Women's Way's responsibility to the agencies is clearly defined; in turn, the agencies will not solicit businesses or individuals, will turn over their individual donor list to become part of the Women's Way list and will conduct only one fundraising event annually. Accountability to Women's Way is ensured through a peer review process which examines management, accounting, financial resource base, and composition and numbers of women served.

The money is divided evenly among the member agencies; each agency is entitled to receive up to 30 percent of the prior year's expenditure. This is based on several premises: (1) all agencies are equal in need; (2) all participate equally in the Women's Way fundraising campaign; (3) Women's Way does not represent the major source of funding for any agency.

Bread and Roses gives annual grants to individual agencies; they can receive only one grant within a 12-month cycle. Although originally Bread and Roses gave the same amount of money to all the grantees, after careful review it shifted to differential funding based on the special needs and capacities of the agency. This shift was suggested to the membership by the executive when it became clear that there were different financial needs and differing access to money among the grantee groups. It was not an easy decision for an organization which had an ideology of cooperating groups and capability of participation, but it was necessary to "bite the bullet."

Bread and Roses has three types of grants: (1) emergency and discretionary, (2) general fund distribution, and (3) donor advised. Grants range from $500 to $5,000.

Black United Fund has two types of allocations: (1) grantee requests, and (2) fund initiated. Thus the Black United Fund is proactive in areas it feels are not being dealt with in the community. For example, it is currently initiating and funding a "Mentor in Business" program to deal with youth unemployment and compatible with the Fund's interest in education and economic development. Grants are made one time only for a specific project; the Fund is careful not to have agencies become too dependent upon it. Grants range in size from $50-$3,000 and are based on in-house resources. Technical assistance and "in-kind" services are also provided.

Both Bread and Roses and Black United Fund expect a follow-up report from the grantee which deals with both the program and financial accountability of each grant.

*(c) Reserve funds* have not been part of the picture for any of the Alternative Funds until recently. This reflects the more affluent position achieved by Women's Way which in 1986 developed a new program goal—"Fund for the Future." The intent is to raise $800,000 for investment purposes. Bread and Roses has also always given all income to the agencies; however, from 1986 it is holding back from $20,000 to $60,000 for reserves. Although Black United Fund is still young and developing, the Board will take a new look at investments for capital funds; until now there have been no reserves.

The decision to develop reserve funds is a critical one which can have the potential of changing the identity of the funds which until now have played a very responsive and flexible role in meeting unorthodox needs. Whether reserves precipitate caution and thus shape the identity of the Alternative Funds will be of concern.

### *(5) Dealing with Controversy*

A careful strategy has been developed to deal with controversial decisions in regard to controversial agencies. This is most clearly delineated by Women's Way since it seeks support from the mainstream community, and from business and industry. Since being pro-choice is a criterion for agency membership in Women's Way, donors who do not wish to support pro-choice activity are allowed to choose funding areas. Funding preferences are honored and this money is removed at the outset, before the regular allocations are made.

Bread and Roses serves a different constituency, whose donors are committed to the fund's social change goals. However, it has modified its position over time; whereas originally a clearly articulated radical analysis was expected in the proposals, this is no longer true. Ideology has given way to performance; the emphasis is on what agencies do.

Black United Fund has a broad service agenda; its donors are committed to service to the black community and the issue of controversial projects is not of concern.

It is clear that Alternative Funds must continuously question the consequences of their activity and do strategic planning in regard to attracting and retaining support of their target donor populations.

*(6) Intrasystem Relations*

Although each of the agencies discussed in this paper developed autonomously, and each has its unique mission and mandate, it is not possible to understand the local system without a broader understanding of the relationships each fund has with the other.

These Alternative Funds are part of a network, both nationally and locally. The national networks serve an array of functions including technical assistance, training and skill development, policy assistance, and professional support to their local units. It is not unexpected that the local units would be closely involved with their parent/national network.

However, one would not expect the diverse local Alternative Funds to be involved actively with one another since one would assume that competitiveness for scarce resources would create a rivalry among them. It is difficult enough for well-funded social programs to work effectively together, let alone programs which are less than secure and stable. And yet, the Philadelphia agencies are actively involved with one another as they plan and strategize together. The prevailing assumption appears to be that what benefits one Alternative Fund benefits all.

This approach did not evolve by chance; it is due to the existence of the Center for Responsible Funding, whose role is a central and critical one. The Center's role as a coordinator is recognized, appreciated and accepted by the three funds. The capacity of this advocacy group to be one step removed from the direct funding mechanisms allows it not only to advocate freely for this alternative system but also to develop strategies which can benefit all the members of the system.

> The Center has also been able to bring together potentially competitive agencies. In the Spring of 1982, the Center convened the first meeting of the Roundtable. Composed of Bread and Roses Community Fund, Women's Way, the Black United Fund of Pennsylvania, and the Combined Health Appeal of the Delaware Valley, the Roundtable meets periodically to discuss matters of common interest and to share information. The group has been able to develop a high degree of cooperation on the City campaign. Its existence has reduced dramatically the level of suspicion and completition among those groups and they look forward to gaining access to other area employers in a cooperative fashion in 1983. (CRF Report, 1982)

The ultimate fruition of these efforts is the existence of a Combined City Campaign for Human Services as well as the School Employees Combined Campaign in which Alternative Funds are included. The Center for Responsible Funding represents the Alternative Funds in the management of these campaigns. (Additional information concerning the technical aspects of the funding approaches may be obtained from the author.)

## *SUMMARY AND IMPLICATIONS*

The legacy of the sixties has been discussed by Levitan (1969) who noted the impact of citizen participation in the human services. Of equal impact is the shaking up of the traditional relationships in the social service sector, relationships which had been rather stable since the turn of the century. Of interest here is the emergence not only of new and progressive agencies seeking social redress and social change, but also new funding mechanisms in the form of Alternative Funds.

The development of an Alternative Fund is indeed a complex phenomenon. Of heuristic value is the experience of the Philadelphia agencies. Critical aspects are highlighted as follows.

First, and perhaps foremost, is the clarity of the organizational mission and the values which define it. What is the unique, distinctive problem to be solved which is not being addressed elsewhere?

Second, a commitment to democratic participation is a unique characteristic of these programs as governance mechanisms are creatively designed. A fundamental assumption of involvement reflects "stake and interest" on the part of the participants, and a nonelitist model obtains.

Third, the resource strategy is carefully developed and reflects the ideological base; thus, it deals not only with obtaining funds, but also the allocations process. A diversified base of support is sought not only to assure fiscal stability but also organizational independence and integrity. In relation to allocations, the grantee agency must demonstrate its capacity not to be totally dependent on the Alternative Fund.

Fourth, controversy is an ongoing fact of life for Alternative Funds, and strategies are needed to anticipate and deal with these situations.

Fifth, the network of nontraditional agencies serves an essential function in terms of support, validation and advocacy. "The more, the merrier" appears to be advantageous, as activity is heightened and more visible.

Sixth, the advocacy function is enhanced by the existence of The Center for Responsible Funding, an organization which serves the Alternative Funds but is not itself a direct funding body.

And last, but not least, the professional leadership of the organizations appears to be far superior to the talent that such remuneration would command in the open market. The executives are ready to make a commitment of time and energy to help these programs remain vital and successful.

It is thus obvious that the development and establishment of an Alternative Fund is a sophisticated and demanding process. The rewards, however, are substantial.

## NOTE

1. Special acknowledgment and appreciation are due to the Executive Directors of those four organizations that gave generously of their time and data: Ann Doley, Bread and Roses; Linda W. Richardson, Black United Fund; Nancy L. Steketee, Center for Responsible Funding; and Lynn H. Yeakel, Women's Way. All case material is taken from the agency documents, questionnaires, and interviews completed by the Executive Directors. Responsibility for the analyses and interpretations rest with the author.

## REFERENCES

Baltzell, D.E. *Philadelphia gentlemen: The making of a national upper class*. New York: Free Press, 1958.

Bothwell, R.O. *United way does not work for all of us*. Washington, DC: National Committee for Responsive Philanthropy, March, 1978.

Cook, R.V. *Activist's guide for organizing an alternative fund*. Washington, DC: National Committee for Responsive Philanthropy, May, 1983.

Davis, K.E. *Fundraising in the black community: History, feasibility and conflict*. Metuchen, NJ: The Scarecrow Press, 1975.

Levitan, S. *The great society's poor law: A new approach to poverty*. Baltimore: Johns Hopkins Press, 1969.

Lubove, R. *The professional altruist*. Cambridge: Harvard University Press, 1965.

Perlmutter, F.D. Public funds and private agencies. *Child Welfare*, 1971, *50*, 264-270.

Perlmutter, F.D. A theoretical model of social agency development. *Social Casework*, 1969, *50*, 467-473.

Seeley, J., et al. *Community chest*. Toronto: University of Toronto Press, 1957.

Selznick, P. *Leadership in administration*. New York: Harper & Row, 1957.

Steiner, J.E. *Community organization: A study of its theory and current practice*. New York: Century Company, 1925.

Teltsch, K. Changing patterns in donations challenge united way methods. *New York Times*, March 8, 1985.

Teltsch, K. Charity dispute splits two funds. *New York Times*, June 13, 1984.

Weisner, S. Fighting back: A critical analysis of coalition building in the human services. *Social Service Review*, 1983, *57*, 291-306.

Wenocur, S., Cook, R.V., & Steketee, N.L. Fund raising at the workplace. *Social Policy*, 1984, *11*, 55-60.

Wilensky, H.L., & Lebeaux, C.N. *Industrial society and social welfare*. New York: Russell Sage Foundation, 1958.

# Administering Alternative Social Agencies: Educational Implications

Felice Davidson Perlmutter, PhD

A broad array of alternative social agencies has been created in the 1970s and 1980s, organized to meet new social needs and to serve populations not eligible for existing social programs in either the public or voluntary sectors (Powell, 1986). The articles in this volume illustrate the breadth of this new system as they describe both direct services and indirect services, and their existence in both the public and the voluntary sectors.

Leadership in these organizations merits special attention since these systems are neither traditionally organized nor traditionally managed. Implications for the administration of these agencies have been addressed elsewhere (Perlmutter, 1988). In this article we will explore the implications for professional education for these roles, based on the assumption that social work is an appropriate professional base for the preparation for leadership in these alternative social agencies.

This article is organized as follows: First, we will highlight the essential characteristics of alternative organizations as presented in this volume; Second, we will suggest leadership characteristics appropriate for these settings; Third, we will discuss implications for curriculum design, including both class and field content in graduate programs. This discussion will be clarified through the use of case material from the papers in this volume.

---

Dr. Perlmutter is Professor, School of Social Administration, Temple University, Philadelphia, PA 19122.

 

## *CHARACTERISTICS OF ALTERNATIVE SOCIAL AGENCIES*

Traditional social agencies in the voluntary sector should welcome the formation of new alternative agencies since they have in common the fact that they were all organized to meet a social need of populations not being adequately served elsewhere in society. As older organizations have matured and stabilized, they have often become sufficiently inflexible and static so that they cannot readily adapt to serve new populations and/or new needs (Perlmutter, 1969). Not only does this serve to accentuate the differences between traditional and alternative agencies, but other differences can also be noted, as follows:

First, alternative agencies are deeply *committed to social change*; not only are they concerned with change in the larger society, but they are equally committed to ideals of participatory democracy, including power equalization and influence (McMahon, 1976). Thus, the Elizabeth Blackwell Health Center for Women has as its mission not only the provision of services to women which are not readily available in the traditional health care system, but of equal importance is its advocacy role, particularly in regard to choice in the matter of abortions. Public education and advocacy are central to the mission of several of the other programs described in the volume, including the Women Reaching Women Project which advocates on behalf of victims of alcoholism and other drug abuse (Kravetz & Jones) and the alternative federated funds which are explicit in their support of agencies committed to social change (F. D. Perlmutter).

Second, alternative agencies *focus on governance structures* with special attention paid to the use of power and hierarchy. Gummer's chapter addresses these issues as he contrasts the structure of traditional service organizations with the new alternative institutions. These issues are also of central concern to Weil, and Schwartz, Gottesman and Perlmutter.

Third, alternative programs are organized to meet the needs of *special populations* with special problems that are not addressed by agencies in the traditional social service sector (Fabricant, 1986). This is clearly illustrated by Shanti which serves people with AIDS and also by the Boone County Community Council which was pushed to include minorities as members of its various commissions.

Fourth, the provision of *new and or innovative services* is discussed in many of the chapters. Fishman's discussion focuses on an administrative structure which is designed to make possible the programmatic implementation of innovative ideas; Blackwell's artificial insemination program for unmarried heterosexual women and lesbians may best illustrate service innovation.

Fifth, *personnel* who staff these programs are certainly not the usual professionals found in health and human services. The primary characteristics of personnel in alternative programs are twofold: They are either themselves members of the target population being served, or ideologically committed to or identified with this population. Thus, a mainstay of each of the direct service programs described in this volume is its volunteers; furthermore the professionals in these organizations serve out of commitment and concern since the traditional benefits of status, money, or power are not available.

Sixth, these organizations view *smallness of size* as an important variable since it permits face to face interaction among all of its participants, a value prized in relation to participatory management. The chapters on Blackwell, Shanti, and Hospice illustrate this commitment.

And seventh, alternative agencies are constantly struggling with their finances since traditional funding approaches are not available to them. Perlmutter's discussion of alternative funds deals most directly with the *resourcing strategies* which have been effective for this special population of agencies.

These seven special attributes must be considered in the design of an educational program which meets the unique needs and interests of alternative social agencies. Before we address the educational implications, it is important to examine the characteristics appropriate for leadership in these systems.

## *LEADERSHIP CHARACTERISTICS FOR ALTERNATIVE AGENCIES*

In our view, leadership in alternative agencies requires a special set of characteristics not usually considered in the leadership literature. Personal characteristics take precedence for people in these roles, although organizational and professional qualifications are also of importance (Perlmutter, 1988).

Personal characteristics are given precedence in order to emphasize the fact that leaders in these agencies must be unconventional; not only must they be imbued with the ideological orientations of the organizations being served, but they must be risk-takers since alternative agencies are highly unstable environments. Furthermore, these leaders must be comfortable with difference, since many different types of people will be involved in various capacities with alternative agencies. And finally, on a personal level, the leadership must be able to tolerate economic insecurity and instability, since the economic base in these organizations is rarely secure.

On an organizational level, a primary skill must be in serving an advocacy function since the broader system requires constant education vis-à-vis the agency's mission. Related to this advocacy function is the urgent need for continuous fundraising and development work. And last but not least, from an organizational standpoint, is the continuous search for new service responses to meet the mission of the agency and the needs of the target population. Blackwell's continuously evolving service system reflects this characteristic.

Professional qualifications also must be carefully considered. These include an understanding of, and capacity to work with, an organization committed to a participatory governance process; a keen understanding of, and involvement with, social policy and relevant legislation is equally necessary. Interpersonal skills are of particular importance in these small and unstable systems, not only on a one-to-one level but also for group and community work. Furthermore, mediating skills can serve a vital function in the many conflict situations which inevitably arise. The final professional skill to be addressed is in personnel work, which includes recruitment, training, and staff development for a rather unconventional array of personnel who staff these agencies.

It thus is obvious that the requisites for leadership in alternative agencies are complex. It is equally clear that careful thought must be given to an educational program which can appropriately prepare leaders for these systems.

## *DESIGNING AN EDUCATIONAL PROGRAM FOR LEADERSHIP IN ALTERNATIVE AGENCIES*

In considering the design of an appropriate vehicle for educating personnel for leadership positions in alternative service agencies it is essential, at the outset, to make explicit two fundamental dilemmas inherent in this process. First, the program is lodged in a formal bureaucracy, albeit a graduate university program; this assumes compliance with the many rules and regulations inherent in professional programs. Second, professional programs represent traditional, and oft conservative, standards of practice; this suggests that while there is much to be learned, there is also much to be unlearned.

While this article addresses both the academic content and the internship experience in the agency setting, major attention will be paid to a field work curriculum. The discussion is intended to delineate and suggest appropriate content in order to stimulate further thinking and design in the many diverse educational settings; consequently it makes no pretense of inclusiveness.

This author has taken the position that personal characteristics are primary in the executive suite of these agencies, a view that has twofold consequences for the graduate programs which wish to develop specializations in this area. First and foremost is the recognition that recruitment and admissions cannot proceed with business as usual. Special outreach efforts must be implemented in order to attract applicants from a population which might not be attracted to graduate professional programs. And the recruitment effort must be coupled with new, flexible and innovative criteria in regard to the applicants for admission. It becomes important to link these criteria to the personal traits which have been suggested above.

Attention must be paid to the diverse characteristics which include ideological commitments to social needs and concerns, attitudes toward difference, experience in risk-taking and innovation, and a readiness to work in settings with marginal economic security. Since most graduate programs require experience in service delivery in order to be admitted to an administrative specialization, the nature of the applicant's past experience can be helpful in assessing the candidacy. And the bottom line must be the applicant's own personal goals and objectives, as well as the applicant's motivation, for specializing in this arena.

Second, in relation to the personal requirements, is the careful design of curriculum content which formally identifies and contributes to the conceptualization and analysis of the precarious values which underpin alternative programs (Clark, 1956). For example, a course in values and ethics would complement and enhance the ideological commitments of the student. Furthermore, the selection of an alternative agency for the internship experience merits special attention as it can provide learning vis-à-vis risk-taking and also make real the experience of working in a marginally resourced setting.

Organizational characteristics essential for leadership in alternative agencies equally require attention in both the class and field settings. Courses should be offered such as budgeting for nonprofit agencies, resource development, fund-raising, the design of management information systems, program design and development, and governance, policy-making, and work with boards. These are some of the skills needed for organizational maintenance in all settings but especially in alternative settings, which must be constantly garnering new support while conserving the scarce resources they command.

The field work setting must be carefully designed to assure not only exposure to, but responsibility for, tasks in these areas. For example, students can be responsible for identifying new funding opportunities, for preparing and writing proposals for funding, for doing needs assessments in relation to new populations and services, for preparation and presentation of testimony of legislative hearings. The underlying premise vis-à-vis the internship experience is that students must have the opportunity to perform in the various areas essential to agency survival which not only contribute to the agency's needs but prepare the students for executive performance.

Professional characteristics must receive equal attention both in academic setting and in the field. Formal course content in participatory democracy and self-management are a *sine qua non* for governance in alternative agencies. Social policy analysis and skills in negotiation and mediation are equally important content areas; and the area of staff recruitment, staff development, and training must also be noted. These content areas lend themselves comfortably to field work assignments, as students must have hands-on experience in policy analysis, staff development, and training.

It is clear that preparation for leadership of alternative agencies is multi-faceted and lends itself comfortably to learning both in the classroom setting and in the field. The dual focus on theory and applications must underpin all content areas. And the educational institution must take the responsibility for the design of the internship experience which will assure that the student is exposed to, and responsible for, quality performance in the field work setting.

The School of Social Administration of Temple University (1987) has designed a field work curriculum which spells out its expectations for the agency placement. The curriculum specifies eight areas in which performance is expected; these include: (1) governance and policy development, (2) program development, (3) personnel administration, (4) supervision and staff development, (5) financial management, (6) funding and resource development, (7) evaluation and control, and (8) interorganizational and public relations. In addition to specifying these areas of expertise, the manual provides a list of suggested assignments in each area which can serve to stimulate new field work strategies appropriate to the agency setting or which can serve as a model for the students' assignments.

Examples of suggested assignments are as follows:

*GOVERNANCE AND POLICY MAKING*

Acquisition of clear understanding of the structure for governance and how policy is made in the agency.

Acquisition of clear understanding of executive role and functions vis-à-vis the board of directors or other governing body.

Observation of general board meetings or board committee meetings.

Other direct or indirect opportunities for participation in policy-making experience.

Preparation and/or presentation of testimony for legislative hearings.

*PROGRAM DEVELOPMENT*

Operationalize goals or objectives for a particular program.

Identify and define resources needed for development of a new program.

Identify legal aspects or implications of new program development.

Assess need for new programming.

Identify staffing pattern required for new program or staffing reorganization required for existing program.

*PERSONNEL ADMINISTRATION*

Review of existing job descriptions; preparation of new job descriptions.

Participation in staff and/or board personnel practices committee meetings.

Preparation of personnel advertisements, recruitment materials.

Screening of job applications; participation in personnel interviewing or hiring procedures.

Review or preparation of orientation materials or orientation program for new staff.

*SUPERVISION, STAFF DEVELOPMENT, AND TRAINING*

Supervision of undergraduate student or other staff personnel.

Review and assess policies regarding continuing education, inservice training, conference attendance, and licensure.

Observe and/or research staff development and/or inservice training program in other agencies.

Develop an inservice training or staff development evaluation tool.

Survey staff regarding wishes or needs for staff development programming.

*FINANCIAL MANAGEMENT*

Comprehend the nature of the budgeting system currently in use in the agency.

Preparation of tentative budget data for next fiscal year:
a) acquisition of relevant and necessary data
b) projection of appropriate values in specific areas

Preparation of tentative program budget framework.

Costing-out of functional area in program budget.

Preparation of reports to funding agencies.

*FUNDING AND RESOURCE DEVELOPMENT*

Identification and investigation of potential new funding streams or opportunities.

Preparation and/or writing of a proposal for new funding or refunding.

Initiation and/or maintenance of communications with funding agencies.

Preparation of reports for funding agencies.

*EVALUATION AND CONTROL*

Needs assessment tasks, in relation to target population.

Analysis of existing information system for compatibility with evaluation needs and/or objectives.

Preparation of materials for professional certification or accreditation reviews, or grant compliance hearing.

Comprehension and/or assessment of administrative control mechanisms in use in agency.

Identification and definition of requirements for feedback information regarding target population, service delivery components, client outcomes, and training outcomes.

*INTERORGANIZATIONAL AND PUBLIC RELATIONS*

Participation in or observation of joint committees to facilitate interagency communication and coordination.

Experience in representing the agency's position to outside agencies and/or groups.

Experience in analyzing the public-private web of services currently and potentially available to meet needs of target population.

Experience in dealing with representatives of the media.

Review or development of overall PR plan for agency or for particular program area.

It must be emphasized that while the educational institution is responsible for the quality and appropriateness of the internship, a participatory process wherein both the agency and the student are partners in the design of the field experience is desirable. Not only does this assure relevance to meet the students' educational needs within the context of agency work which must be done, but it appropriately serves as a model for the participatory process.

## *IN CONCLUSION*

The profile for leadership in alternative social agencies is a complex one; its unique characteristics must be nurtured and protected. As noted earlier, there are special dilemmas inherent in training for that leadership in a traditional professional educational program, and careful attention must be paid to use what is relevant and to cast off what may be dysfunctional. The dangers of professional credentials have been noted in the literature (Glasscote et al., 1975, Gonsiorek, 1982). But to be forewarned is to be forearmed.

In our view, these new agencies require special expertise on the part of their leaders, expertise which can ensure survival without abandoning a unique organizational mission and domain. And this leadership can be developed and nurtured in professional educational programs which can be sensitive to the content which is needed and flexible in the internship which must be designed.

## REFERENCES

Clark, B. R. Organizational adaptation and precarious values. *American Sociological Review*, 1956, *21*, 327-336.

Fabricant, M. Creating survival services. *Administration in Social Work*, Fall 1986, *10*, 71-84.

Glasscote, R.M., Raybin, J.B., Reifler, C.B., & Kane, A.W. *The alternative services: Their role in mental health*. Washington, DC: American Psychiatric Association, 1975.

Gonsiorek, J.C. Organizational and staff problems in gay/lesbian mental health agencies. *Journal of Homosexuality*, 1982, *7*, 193-208.

McMahon, J.T. Participation and power equalized organizational systems. *Human Relations*, 1976, *29*, 203-214.

Perlmutter, F.D. Administering alternative social programs. In L. Ginsberg & P. Keys (Eds.), *Modern management and social work*. Silver Spring, MD: NASW, 1988.

Perlmutter, F.D. A theoretical model of social agency development. *Social Casework*, 1969, *50*, 467-473.

Powell, D.M. Managing organizational problems in alternative service agencies. *Administration in Social Work*, Fall 1986, *10*, 57-69.

Temple University School of Social Administration. *Field work curriculum*, 1987. Unpublished school/agency curriculum statement.

# PART 4: EPILOGUE

Albert E. Wilkerson, DSW

The creation of alternative human service agencies, while not a totally new phenomenon, brings certain new dimensions to the field. First, they are now sufficient in number as to be recognized as a distinct movement. Second, they institutionalize a basic social reform theme: It is not necessarily the established power-brokers and/or the professionals who will determine what the client group needs and how the services will be delivered. And third, the movement is of ample size and import to be not only a competition threat but also a resource of innovations for infusion into the traditional service models.

The purpose of this volume has been to present a sample of the diversity of the alternative responses to urgent and sensitive problems and issues, to encourage self-assessment within the movement, and to begin to identify for the field those perceptions, inputs, and processes that make for success or lead to failure; and, in so doing, to contribute to bringing to both professional and public awareness lagging opportunities and social obligations.

In the beginning phases, service directions in our field are experimental, evolving out of a response to human necessity or fresh social themes. Then follow formative assessment, empirical research, and program correction. The contributing authors were asked to examine agency philosophy, structure, policies, and protocols. Not surprisingly, with agencies possessing virtually identical philosophy and goals, overwhelming similarities follow in other organizational aspects.

---

Dr. Wilkerson is Professor, School of Social Administration, Temple University, Philadelphia, PA 19122. He also serves as Assistant Editor of *Administration in Social Work*.

 

The current phase of continued experimentation and assessment is promising, with its successes and anticipations, but it also provides clues as to possible pitfalls. In reflecting upon appropriate themes for an Epilogue for this volume, which moves through description and into initial analysis, it is these anticipations versus pitfalls that come boldly into view.

## *WHY ALTERNATIVE HUMAN SERVICE AGENCIES?*

Alternative human service agencies emerge when there is a perception by an interest group that the existing institutional objectives, service structures, and program content cannot, or will not, be quickly and appropriately responsive to special client populations.

This perception is a serious critique of the human services enterprise in that it challenges basic images that traditional organizations hold about themselves. It does not trust that the enterprise is essentially innovative, flexible, and generous. It views professionals as trapped in the rigid, sluggish, and self-serving nature of bureaucracy. And, it holds to the view that a given client population has needs so special as to make current approaches inadequate or obsolete.

Such a critique thus gives rise to the necessity for a different approach – a new organizational form, a new pattern of organizational behaviors, and a new set of staff-client interactions. In one sense, the objective is to create something "unique" for "special" clients. In another, it is to revive and enhance longstanding, uncorrupted service ideals: a generosity of outreach, whatever the human plight; a practice that represents the best human relations principles; and form and climate that ensure client self-determination and participation, and that are infused with democracy for staff.

In another facet, they are an example of how, in an affluent society, we can afford to set up parallel systems to do the job that an existing system is failing to do.

An essential building block in alternative agencies is a holdover from a popular and professional belief that emerged strongly during the recent reform period – that the most effective understanding and assistance are provided by persons (former clients or professionals) who have experienced the condition personally or who share with the clientele some other problem-related bond.

Uniqueness, creativity, innovation, democracy, equality, service responsiveness, client involvement, advocacy, and, more recently, empowerment, are words that form rather uniform battle cries across the human services field. But, the individual and organizational tendencies toward self-serving and self-perpetuating behaviors, the predictable slide toward bureaucratic stultification, and the absence of sufficient evaluations of program effectiveness, pit the positives and negatives against one another with what seems to be an unfailing rhythm and intensity.

Against the bureaucratic norm, the alternative human service agency is a cleansing of the air, a new ambiance, and a fresh hope that as professionals we can be above the organizational entrapments that short-circuit our humanitarian purposes. They make us feel unshackled, unselfish, free, and genuinely responsive to our mission. They are re-energizing and filled with positive anticipation.

But, within the context of classical organizational theory, there are certain problems inherent within such a movement, with implications in the areas of organizational survival, the executive's leadership role, and social policy development.

## ORGANIZATIONAL ISSUES

### The Life Cycle of Charismatic Organizations

The character of alternative human service agencies has been observed readily as charismatic in nature. The essentials of charismatic organizations, as identified by Weber (in Gerth & Mills, Eds., 1946; Parsons et al., Eds., 1965) and elaborated upon by Blau and Scott (1962), Merton (1957), Parsons (1960), and Etzioni (1961, 1969) are: a leadership of magnetic qualities; an adherence to a belief system that approaches religiosity; a process of staff acculturation that separates "insiders" from "outsiders"; and a protocol that uniformly regulates professional and organizational behaviors.

Students of charismatic organizations and movements also have identified certain pitfalls in such phenomena. These pitfalls appear to be inherent, marking a rather predictable life cycle that eventually comes to an end through attrition. Gummer recalls three kinds of alternative human service agencies earlier described by Seeley et al. (1957). They are: a "poor copy" of the idealized; a "complementary system," akin to an ancillary function; and the "contradiction," a statement of negation of existing forms. It must be readily apparent that the poor copy and the contradiction are those most at risk.

The leaders successive to the founder are credited with the same attributes and capabilities of the founder, whether or not in reality they possess them. If they do possess them, the life of the movement is more easily extended. But, should this imputation be based on incorrect assessment, cracks in the system quickly appear. Should the new leader prove to be either less than expected or to have too many different ideas, and thus does not really fit the mold, the followers quickly become anxious, suspicious, and rebellious.

As the belief system crystallizes and takes on an aura of sacredness, a litany of thought and behaviors follows, from which no one wishes, or dares, to deviate. A sacred belief system has its advantages. Behavior is committed and easily predictable, and the work processes tend to run smoothly. Irrational decisions (i.e., self-centered agendas) are kept to a minimum, since the oneness of the group serves as a continuous monitor and corrective force.

Over time, the foundation blocks and original intellectual sources for the belief system become blurred. With the past blurred, present behavior becomes automatic. New ideas become anathemas. Changes seem disloyal. The leaders become less charming. The heir selected by a charismatic leader may be chosen for one's unwavering loyalty and obeisance rather than for capability. Essentially, such an heir is expected to play a caretaker role. (Weil describes a more fortunate situation in which the two successive executives were clearly atypical of this kind of succession problem.) The charismatic organization normally dies a natural death by withering away from a lack of a continuous flow of nutrients. The "New Beginnings" project described by Fishman gives an advantage by providing a continuous flow of new service directions within a constant belief system and form.

The secret to life-extension lies, then, in a carefully controlled leadership succession, in controlled acculturation of staff, in exclusion of persons whose nature is to challenge, and yet in being able to reexamine and modify philosophy and practice as the times change, without wavering from the central purpose. Unfortunately, the very effort toward flexibility corrupts the singular agreement as to purpose, form, and content. In this attempt to survive the times and trends, the most enthusiastic charismatic organization probably will yield to the bureaucratic model. Weber referred to this natural tendency as "the routinization of charisma" (reprinted in Parsons et al., 1965).

### Process versus Client Outcomes

Alternative human service agencies, because of their charismatic and egalitarian nature, spend an inordinate amount of effort on process: process in staff hiring, acculturation, and evaluation; process in budget allocations; process in peer supervision; process in conflict resolution; etc.

An emphasis on process is necessary in order to carry out the avowed goals of this type of agency and should serve to enhance consistency in organizational purpose, to ensure uniformity in staff behaviors, and to increase effective client outcomes.

There is no doubt that process can seem to be energizing, even exhilarating. A feeling of oneness, a clarity in performance guides, a workplace that values personal significance, and a strong group support, are all positives. But the repayment to the organization is through extensive committee work, complex decision-making mechanisms, and a continuous preserving and defending the belief system—all while involved in the negotiating, compromising, and testing one's own status, the activities that occur in every workplace.

The problem, of course, is a matter of time and energy. Democracy in agency affairs, a concept intensified by the social reform movement, must shift both time and energy from outcome to process. When this occurs, the client gets what remains after internal business has taken its physical and psychological tolls. Hooyman, Fredriksen, and B. Perlmutter note the very delicate "balance between process and task performance" in the work of staff, and particularly of volunteers. Stultifying as it may be, a bureaucratic model relieves staff of many of these time-consuming and energy-draining activities. The choice of one model over the other involves trade-offs. But with the trade-offs, both models possess the seeds for demoralization and burn-out.

Alternative human service agencies, however, are nearer to an ideal functioning and must be valued for their intent. The potential pitfall lies in whether or not there are adequate controls to prevent process from deflecting too much from attention to client-outcome, as it is very easy to equate staff process (form and method) with agency productivity. This poses a significant area for more intensive study in both organizational theory and outcome evaluation.

### *The Tenuous Nature of External Funding*

A third survival issue, as also noted in the present collection of papers, relates to the necessity for a stable and continuous funding flow. Funding sources follow the emergence of front-burner social issues and crises. Governmental, foundation, and corporate-giving programs all have a bent toward a somewhat whimsical nature: When a more attractive or urgent social need attracts their attention, or when social themes change—due to politics, economics, or new social threats—the money route can move in a mercurial flow, contributing to the typically short life-span of the alternative human service agency.

Felice Perlmutter has focused upon alternative federated funding as a mechanism which responds to new or alternative human services in an effort to bypass idiosyncratic and conservative giver-motives. Despite the common interests and goals of the alternative human service agencies, the competitive factor in the search for dollars remains strong. Indeed, the creation of alternative agencies obviously has increased the competition among service providers and, as she points out, has increased the rivalry among them. Fee-for-service is used by some agencies not only to generate income but also as an effort to avoid program controls that might be imposed through grants.

The continuing financial crisis within the human services enterprise should prompt a more concerted effort by both traditional and alternative agencies to create more structured and vigorous development functions within the organizations, either individually or in consortia arrangements. The "development function" here specifically means an office of "financial resourcing."

The sources for financial resourcing within a full development program include not only the standard federated funding sources and proposal entries for project grants from governmental agencies, foundations, and corporations, but also the creating of a strong support group that can assist in an extensive program in major fund-raising events and all aspects of planned philanthropy. Such a dynamic development function can be modeled after the successes of numerous cultural, educational, and health-related institutions.

## THE EXECUTIVE'S ROLE DILEMMA

"Leadership" and "authority" are implicit role concepts in organizational titles such as "Director," "Executive Director," "President," and "Chief Executive Officer." In a horizontal management arrangement, the line between coordinating and attending to maintenance functions and asserting leadership and authority is by design ambiguous. It appears that this ambiguity is dealt with in alternative human service agencies by a group consensus which establishes a buffer zone wide enough to absorb a significant degree of group floundering; and, when the edge is finally reached, the exercise of administrative leadership and authority is welcomed and thus normally not challenged.

It is the charismatic nature of alternative human service agencies that allows for such mobile boundaries. The leader is clearly accepted as "first among equals"; but, there can be a fairly wide difference between the "first" member and the other members either individually or as a whole. The charismatic leader, with the attribution of unusual human qualities, is able to exert a certain will to which the group assents rather easily. This act of acquiescence psychologically moves very quickly to making the leader's will the group will, so that the leader's ideas and enactments can be easily felt as group decisions and actions, as long as they are within the accepted boundaries of organizational purpose and spirit. Thus, the dilemma in the non-exercise of implicit role requirements for an executive is dissolved by the power of the leader's real or imputed charm.

More difficult administrative dilemmas must lie, however, in other kinds of staff behaviors, interactions, expectations, and ambitions that are certain to exist in both bureaucratic and horizontal organizations.

Staff "equals" do not tend to stay equal indefinitely. There are over-achievers and under-achievers, the less assertive and the more assertive, the less competent and the more competent, those temporarily holding their own agendas in check and those who are by nature more organizationally oriented, and those who are essentially self-effacing and those who ultimately will look around for rewards and perks. And, there is generally a self-appointed heir, who is making moves in a determined direction. Juggling within these sets of human dynamics and variables, that are bound to develop, must be the most delicate of tasks, and it is no doubt here that the charisma of the executive is most strenuously put to test.

In such situations, the dynamics finally become self-centered; and the group fervor that characteristically carries the flow of democracy, enthusiasm, and compliance ultimately breaks. How many minor cracks can be sustained and whether they can be repaired in an alternative human service agency, short of moving to the bureaucratic model, is an intriguing area for more experimentation and investigation. Current theory is skeptical.

## *SOCIAL POLICY IMPLICATIONS*

There was a time in human services work when the idea of a "recovered client" as helper was dismally viewed by professionals. The recovered client, in addition to the probability of inadequate training/education, was viewed as bringing an idiosyncratic, or lopsided, view to the helping effort. The reform movement reversed the traditional opinion; and for a period of time there was enormous emphasis placed upon a belief in an unusual effectiveness of the recovered client's abilities. When the helper was not a "recovered client," there were at least certain bonds held in common (e.g., race, sex, age, social and ethnic backgrounds, etc.) that were presumed to be of prime significance in understanding and helping the other. At present, there seems to be a more balanced perception concerning such potential and inappropriateness.

The idea of like-mindedness as a helping dynamic is based in a belief that there is something so "special" about a given phenomenon that only the sufferers can really comprehend it and respond correctly to it. While there is some logical defense for this, particularly at major turning points in the history of the problem, a coopting of the problem rests on a foundation theory that is essentially faulty.

Alternative human service agencies, in the core of their belief systems, smack of this faulty theory. These new arrangements are responses to target populations victimized by general public neglect, under-funded service provisions, and even broad-based societal distaste and prejudice. The potential pitfall lies in whether or not the agencies and organizations will be able to give up the idea of the "special" nature of their clientele at an appropriate point and encourage mainstream service organizations to provide services as a natural response to a human problem.

Given the nature of charismatic organizations and the enthusiasm and protectiveness of those championing a cause, along with the label of special or different, the alternative human service agency might, in the long run, impede the rate of societal response by keeping the target population too long out of the pale of normative human services.

Alcoholics Anonymous, despite its successes as a long-surviving charismatic organization, does a certain disservice to its members. Its belief that only a recovered alcoholic can be useful to another, its belief that the organization's protocol is the only correct one, its adherence to a far outdated "allergy" theory, its antagonism toward psychological theory and research findings, and its ambivalence toward medical supports, have for decades made the alcoholic and alcoholism so "special" a case that the various helping and treatment professions have largely stayed away from the problem.

To avoid this potential pitfall, the alternative human service agency should have a strong advocacy component within its current program, with an aim to reduce public prejudice, increase positive community interest, influence rational social policy, and assist mainstream service agencies to create and/or expand services for the clientele for whom they are now doing the groundwork by highlighting and being creatively responsive. Schwartz, Gottesman, and F.D. Perlmutter, among others writing in this volume, have emphasized the agency's very deliberate dual priority on "both social change and internal organizational structure."

The emergence of the alternative human service agency is an important development in the helping professions for two main reasons: They reflect an idealized organizational character and protocol; and they intend to offer a maximum service to the clientele. Such an organization is no doubt possible only when its purpose is nonprofit, as long as its leader possesses a certain set of personality attributes, and as long as a skilled staff can remain focused upon the client rather than upon self.

The study of alternative human service agencies is at present in the descriptive and self-assessment stages. Outcome studies and empirical research, the emphases needed for the immediate future, will provide data and guides as to how these agencies can survive at least long enough to place their causes largely on the map, influence social policy development, and spark a broad-based direct service response from the community.

## REFERENCES

Blau, P.M., & Scott, W.R. *Formal organizations: A comparative approach*. San Francisco: Chandler Publishing Co., 1962.

Etzioni, A. *A comparative analysis of complex organizations*. New York: The Free Press of Glencoe, 1961.

Etzioni, A. *A sociological reader on complex organizations*. Second edition. New York: Holt, Rinehart and Winston, 1969.

Merton, R.K. *Social theory and social structure*. Revised edition. Glencoe, IL: The Free Press, 1957.

Parsons, T. *Structure and process in modern societies*. Glencoe, IL: The Free Press, 1960.

Seeley, J.R., et al. *Community chest: A case study in philanthropy*. Toronto: University of Toronto Press, 1957.

Weber, M. Bureaucracy. In H.H. Gerth & C.W. Mills (Eds.), *From Max Weber: Essays in sociology*. New York: Oxford University Press, 1946.

Weber, M. The routinization of charisma. In T. Parsons, et al. (Eds.), *Theories of society: Foundations of modern sociological theory*. One volume edition. New York and London: The Free Press of Glencoe, 1965.